Pope Francis and the Transformation of Health Care Ethics

Pope Francis and the Transformation of Health Care Ethics

Todd A. Salzman and Michael G. Lawler

Georgetown University Press / Washington, DC

The publisher is not responsible for third-party websites or their content. URL links were active at time of publication.

Library of Congress Cataloging-in-Publication Data
Names: Salzman, Todd A., author. | Lawler, Michael G., author.
Title: Pope Francis and the transformation of health care ethics / Todd A. Salzman and Michael G. Lawler.
Description: Washington, DC : Georgetown University Press, 2021. | Includes bibliographical references and index.
Identifiers: LCCN 2020023073 | ISBN 9781647120702 (hardcover) | ISBN 9781647120719 (paperback) | ISBN 9781647120726 (ebook)
Subjects: LCSH: Francis, Pope, 1936– | Catholic Church. United States Conference of Catholic Bishops. Ethical and religious directives for Catholic health facilities. | Catholic health facilities. | Medical ethics—Religious aspects—Catholic Church. | Social ethics—Religious aspects—Catholic Church.
Classification: LCC RA975.C37 S25 2021 | DDC 174.2—dc23
LC record available at https://lccn.loc.gov/2020023073

♾ This book is printed on acid-free paper meeting the requirements of the American National Standard for Permanence in Paper for Printed Library Materials.

22 21   9 8 7 6 5 4 3 2 First printing

Printed in the United States of America
Cover design by Nathan Putens
Interior design by Paul Hotvedt, Blue Heron Typesetters

Pope Francis refers to doctors and nurses serving during the coronavirus pandemic as the "saints next door."

This book is dedicated to all the saints who give themselves so selflessly to the care and health of others.

Contents

Abbreviations

AG	*Ad Gentes* (Decree on the Church's Missionary Activity). Second Vatican Council. Vatican City, 1965.
AL	Pope Francis. *Amoris Laetitia* (The Joy of Love). Vatican City, 2016.
ANH	artificial nutrition and hydration
CCC	*Catechism of the Catholic Church.* Vatican City: Libreria Editrice Vaticana, 1993.
CDF	Congregation for the Doctrine of the Faith
DH	*Dignitatis Humanae* (Declaration on Religious Freedom). Second Vatican Council. Vatican City, 1965.
ERD	*Ethical and Religious Directives for Catholic Health Care Services.* Washington, DC: United States Conference of Catholic Bishops, 2018.
EG	Pope Francis. *Evangelii Gaudium* (The Joy of the Gospel). Vatican City, 2013.
FC	Pope John Paul II. *Familiaris Consortio* (Exhortation on the Role of the Christian Family). Vatican City, 1982.
GS	*Gaudium et Spes* (Pastoral Constitution on the Church in the Modern World). Second Vatican Council. Vatican City, 1965.
HV	Pope Paul VI. *Humanae Vitae* (On Human Life). Vatican City, 1968.
LG	*Lumen Gentium* (Dogmatic Constitution on the Church). Second Vatican Council. Vatican City, 1964.
LS	Pope Francis. *Laudato Si'* (On Care for Our Common Home). Vatican City, 2015.
PL	J. P. Migne. *Patrologiae Cursus Completus: Series Latina.*
PVS	persistent vegetative state

SRS   Pope John Paul II. *Sollicitudo Rei Socialis* (The Social Concern of the Church). Vatican City, 1987.

ST   *Summa Theologiae Sancti Thomae de Aquino*

USCCB   United States Conference of Catholic Bishops

VS   John Paul II. *Veritatis Splendor* (The Splendor of Truth). Vatican City, 1993.

All translations from languages other than English are the authors'.

Overview of the *Ethical and Religious Directives for Catholic Health Care Services*

In June 2018 the United States Conference of Catholic Bishops (USCCB) released the sixth edition of the *Ethical and Religious Directives for Catholic Health Care Services (ERD)*. We present a critical commentary on the revised *ERD* focusing on two events, one that should be clearly evident in any revision of the *ERD* that the USCCB would issue, the other more subtle but profoundly impacting the entire Church and the authority, authenticity, and credibility of the bishops individually and collectively. The first event is Pope Francis's papacy, which began on March 13, 2013, five years before the revised *ERD* was published. Francis has fundamentally transformed Catholic anthropology, ecclesiology, and ethical methodology, yet there is no evidence of this transformation in the revised *ERD*. We are guided by the transformative impact of Francis's papacy throughout this commentary and demonstrate how it should impact future revisions of the *ERD* in particular and Catholic health care ethics in general.[1] The second event is the clerical sex-abuse scandal. While the scandal was covered up by *some* bishops, it has fundamentally transformed the authority, credibility, and authenticity of *all* bishops. The revised *ERD* provides no evidence that the USCCB grasps the impact of this crisis on bishops' and the Church's authority and credibility. It continues to emphasize the bishop's authority over health care decisions in his diocese as if his authority and credibility are fully intact and untarnished. We address this issue in detail in chapter 6.

The first edition of the *ERD* was published in 1948, with several subsequent revisions.[2] As science and technology advance, health care delivery becomes more complex; cooperation between Catholic and non-Catholic health care providers further complicates it and raises moral questions on the role and function of institutional Catholic mission and identity. The 2018 edition of the *ERD* is virtually the same as the fifth edition, with the exception of part 6, which has substantial revisions guiding "Collaborative Arrangements with Other Health Care Organizations and Providers." The *ERD* seeks to provide ethical guidelines, grounded in "the natural moral law, Church teaching or canon law" (*ERD*, 23), to guide Catholic institutions in the provision of health care that reflects both the healing ministry of Jesus and his Church's understanding of human dignity.

Since its first edition, numerous academic and pastoral articles have been written on the *ERD*, but there has not been a recent book-length commentary analyzing its directives. The closest scholarly works reflecting such a commentary are a series of five booklets written by Gerald Kelly between 1949 and 1955 titled *Medico-Moral Problems*, a revisionist proposal by Richard McCormick in 1984, and a manual-type commentary by Orville Griese in 1987.[3] The essays from Kelly's booklets were arranged topically to follow the sequence of directives in the second and revised edition of the *ERD* and published in 1958.[4] Kelly was largely responsible for authoring the 1949 and 1956 editions of the *ERD*, and his booklets are more an explanation of the directives than a critical analysis. McCormick's text is a commentary on "Ethical Guidelines for Catholic Health Care Institutions," itself a proposal by Catholic theologians, health care professionals, and ethicists, who responded to the invitation from the 1971 "Ethical and Religious Directives for Catholic Health Facilities" to revise the *ERD* in light of scientific and theological developments.[5] McCormick's text focuses on anthropological, ethical methodological, and ecclesiological developments at the Second Vatican Council and its aftermath that mark a fundamental transition in Catholic theological ethics. Griese began his text with a helpful historical overview of the *ERD* and focused on nine principles that explain and justify the directives and provide a manualistic guide to pastoral and moral practices in Catholic hospitals. We believe it is important to contribute a critical analysis of the most recent edition of the *ERD*, which is in large part a repetition of the 2001 and 2009 editions, for several reasons.

We find the 2018 edition of the *ERD* problematic anthropologically, methodologically, ecclesiologically, and pastorally as well as specifically in its attempt to navigate mergers between Catholic and non-Catholic institutions. Anthropologically, it continues to prioritize a biological over a relational ontology as the foundation for its norms and principles guiding health care, despite the relational shift in Catholic theological ethics since the Second Vatican Council. Methodologically, it has not incorporated recent developments in Catholic theological ethics that have shifted from an act-centered to a virtue-centered method. The focus in the *ERD*, especially with respect to the beginning and the end of life, continues to be on absolute norms that proscribe particular acts. There is also a deficit in the consideration of Catholic social teaching and its integration with Catholic sexual teaching. The broadening of Catholic social teaching and its concerns with race, immigration, refugees, economics, global health, and artificial intelligence evidence the too-narrow vision of the *ERD* and the need to expand it to address the issues and complexity of health care ethics thoughtfully and comprehensively. Catholic social and sexual teachings reflect very different methodologies that demand integration in health care ethics.

Ecclesiologically, past editions of the *ERD* focus on patient, physician, and institutional obedience to magisterial teaching and on the authority of local bishops to make decisions regarding the interpretation and application of the *ERD*. The sixth edition "strengthen[s] the role of the local Bishop" in making those decisions.[6] We believe the emphases on the authority of, and obedience to, the local bishop raise some important ecclesiological questions. First, the emphasis in the *ERD* is on the local bishop and his authority in his diocese. The bishop certainly does have teaching authority ecclesially and canonically, but *how* this authority is exercised in health care ethics, policy, and delivery raises ecclesiological concerns. The authority of the bishop emphasized in the *ERD* too often represents a pre–Second Vatican Council hierarchical ecclesiology that the council replaced with a communion ecclesiology.[7] There is a very narrow recognition of a communion ecclesiology in the *ERD*; its perspective is guided predominantly by a hierarchical ecclesiology. Second, there is no consideration of or appreciation for the *sensus fidelium* as an essential dimension of a communion ecclesiology in the *ERD*. This is a betrayal of Catholic tradition and the ecclesiological vision of the Second Vatican Council. Third, there is no acknowledgment of the sex-abuse crisis or its impact on episcopal authority, credibility, and authenticity individually and collectively. We shall deal with communion ecclesiology and *sensus fidelium* in some detail in chapter 4 and the implications of the sex-abuse crisis for the *ERD* in chapter 6.

In addition, the *ERD* "offers little that is of help to persons seeking to understand the importance and centrality of pastoral/spiritual care in Catholic health care."[8] Jean deBlois appeals to the bishops to read the "signs of the times" regarding the state of Catholic health care and to respond in a deeper and more spiritual way to people's needs. The signs today are remarkably similar to but more complex than the signs she was reading in 2009: religious and ethical pluralism; political, religious, cultural, and moral polarization; economic challenges, especially for the uninsured and underinsured; and the challenges of delivering health care in light of the immigration crisis, which itself begs for compassionate care and redress. These considerations, combined with the reality of a priest shortage and lack of serious theological training for pastoral ministers, demand ecclesial, pastoral, moral, and perhaps even canonical responses.

Finally, in terms of collaboration and mergers between Catholic and non-Catholic institutions, there is a broader ecclesiological issue within the Church in general, and the *ERD* in particular, on how to resolve conflicts between bishops if and when there are disagreements between them on collaboration between Catholic and non-Catholic health care institutions that span across multiple dioceses. As health care delivery becomes more complex and non-Catholic organizations merge with Catholic ones and expand across dioceses and states, there will inevitably continue to be disagreements between bishops about how to interpret and apply the *ERD* in general and the principles of legitimate cooperation in specific. The acknowledgment of such disagreements and criteria for resolving them are vague, both in the *ERD* and in canon law. We propose throughout this commentary that the Catholic way to reconcile such disagreements and differences is the way of dialogue of charity recommended by Popes John Paul II and Francis. Listen, Francis advises: "Keep an open mind. Don't get bogged down in your own limited ideas and opinions but be prepared to change or expand them. The combination of two different ways of thinking can lead to a synthesis that enriches both. The unity we seek is not a uniformity, but a unity in diversity." He goes on in a Church-communion perspective, teaching that "fraternal communion is enriched by respect and appreciation for differences within an overall perspective that advances the common good" (*AL*, 139). His advice should be followed by bishops who disagree about the interpretation and application of the *ERD* and by all Catholics, as we shall see, who disagree about doctrinal or moral issues. Disagreements between bishops and how their authority is to be exercised in disputed moral health care issues is not adequately treated in the 2018 revised *ERD*.

The anthropological, methodological, and ecclesiological issues evident in the 2018 edition of the *ERD*, as well as the challenges of pastoral/spiritual ministry and collaboration between Catholic and non-Catholic institutions, have a historical basis reflected in the evolution of the *ERD* itself. We explore that history, provide an overview of the contents of the current *ERD*, and introduce the most basic metaethical question of ethical discourse to begin our critical analysis of the *ERD*: is there such a thing as ethical truth?

A BRIEF HISTORICAL OVERVIEW OF THE *ERD*

There is a long history of Catholic concern for the care and treatment of the sick and infirm, grounded in Jesus' healing ministry.[9] Catholics believe that

Jesus of Nazareth is God incarnate in the world and that he is "the way, the truth, and the life" to the Father (John 14:6). When they read the Gospel accounts of Jesus' life, they discover that he was both a teacher and a renowned healer and that he passed on this double mission to his apostles, sending them out "to preach the kingdom of God and to heal" (Luke 9:1–2). This mission to preach and to heal is one of the foundations of Catholic health care ministry, and concern about it became more pronounced and deliberate in the sixteenth century and continues to evolve over time.

Issues such as how to determine death and which procedures were necessary or optional to prolong life were often discussed. No formal guidelines were issued early on, but priest-theologians did develop general norms for the care and treatment of patients. As Catholic religious communities began to focus more on health care and Catholic hospitals became more prevalent in the late nineteenth and early twentieth centuries in Canada and the United States, there was a recognized need for the systematic formulation of norms and guidelines for both Catholic health care practitioners and institutions to ensure effective patient care and to protect the rights of Catholic hospitals and health care facilities. To those ends, the Catholic Hospital Association (CHA; later named the Catholic Health Association) was established in 1915. The CHA recognized the importance of issuing guidelines to address difficult moral issues in the delivery of health care. The first set of guidelines was formulated by Michael Burke for the Archdiocese of Detroit in 1921 and focused on surgical procedures such as direct sterilization or destruction of fetal life. This was a one-page list of norms that was modified in some cases and posted on the walls of operating rooms in many US and Canadian Catholic hospitals.

The rule-oriented guidelines stated the "dos and don'ts" of surgical procedures deemed most controversial at the time but offered no theological foundation. As health care evolved and the moral issues involved in its delivery became more complex, there was a recognized need for standardizing the guidelines and articulating a foundation and structure to justify them. Theologians and health care professionals began work on this project in 1947, and in 1948 the *Ethical and Religious Directives for Catholic Hospitals (ERD)* was published. It was not a mandatory code for Catholic hospitals to follow, but its adoption was subject to the discretion of the local bishop. Many bishops in Canada and the United States did adopt it. After World War II, Canada instituted universal health care, and, since this system had a very different form of delivery with distinct ethical issues from the United States, Canadian hospitals, under the supervision of the Canadian bishops, thereafter established their own Catholic health care association. In 1954 the Canadian bishops adopted the *Code of Ethical Directives* for Catholic hospitals in their dioceses. In the United States the *ERD* was revised and expanded in 1956 to make it more accessible to Catholic hospitals and health care practitioners. The revision sought both to be more systematic and user friendly, including an index and reference material, and to address broader issues like professional confidentiality, pastoral and spiritual ministry to non-Catholics, and psychological treatment.

Jesuit moral theologian Gerald Kelly was the principal author of the 1949 and 1956 directives. He published a number of articles explaining and commenting on the directives in the journal *Hospital Progress* (now *Health Progress*), which were collected and later published in the first comprehensive commentary on the *ERD*.[10] The various editions of the *ERD* were published to give clear moral guidelines and consistent interpretation of those guidelines for Catholic health care facilities. It continued to be acknowledged that the local bishop was ultimately responsible for its adoption, interpretation, and application. Interpretation of the *ERD* was rather uniform in the 1950s and early 1960s, but with the development of the new ethical method of proportionalism among Catholic moral theologians, the directives began to be interpreted divergently on issues such as contraception and sterilization, depending on whether the local bishop was progressive or conservative. Proportionalism is an ethical method that discerns the premoral values and disvalues of an act to judge whether the premoral value can justify causing the premoral disvalue in any given act. Proportionate reason is used to facilitate this judgment. Progressive bishops recognized the contribution of this principle, which is established in Catholic tradition and frequently cited in the *ERD* itself, especially on end-of-life treatment decisions, to guide health care professionals and patients in making responsible ethical decisions. Conservative bishops used the principle of proportionate reason in end-of-life issues to determine the benefits and burdens of treatment, but they rejected its relevance on other issues, such as contraception and sterilization.[11] Different episcopal interpretations of the *ERD* led to what we may call "geographical morality," morality that depends on the location of the hospital and of the bishop interpreting the *ERD*. These different interpretations point to different methodological perspectives that have profound implications for the interpretation and application of the *ERD*, depending on whether a bishop is conservative or progressive. This tension is amplified, as we discuss in detail in chapter 7, by Catholic and non-Catholic mergers that span several dioceses where there are several Catholic hospitals, like those owned by Catholic Health Initiative, and different diocesan bishops who oversee the hospitals and the interpretation and application of the *ERD* within them.

In response to "geographical morality" and to standardize the interpretation and application of the *ERD*, the CHA Board of Trustees requested the National Conference of Catholic Bishops (NCCB), now the United States

Conference of Catholic Bishops, to formulate and promulgate a uniform set of *ERD* for the United States. Such a standardization, CHA hoped, would eliminate geographical morality. In 1971 a new *ERD* was published with overwhelming support from the bishops, though many theologians had theological and ethical concerns. The 1971 *ERD* was legalistic in its approach and did not offer any theological rationale or justification for its directives, merely stating them as rules to be followed. As we shall see, there were and are anthropological and methodological tensions in the *ERD* when comparing different directives. There was, however, a sense of urgency for the bishops to promulgate this edition of the *ERD* before the coming US Supreme Court ruling on *Roe v. Wade* (1973), which legalized abortion, and injunctions by federal courts rejecting prohibitions of sterilizations in Catholic hospitals. Cardinal John Krol of Philadelphia, president of the NCCB at the time, pushed for adoption of the *ERD* by bishops throughout the United States so that they would be on record as forbidding these and other procedures judged to violate "religious teaching." It was believed that the federal conscience clause would protect Catholic health care facilities and professionals when they refused to perform these procedures. The new *ERD* did not eliminate the threat of geographical morality, especially on issues like sterilization to prevent a future pathology.

The legalistic nature of the 1971 *ERD* and the lack of methodological and theological justification for it, as well as emerging moral issues such as the need for informed consent for research subjects, led to another revision of the *ERD*. Taking advice from theologians, moralists, medical practitioners, and its own committee on doctrine, the NCCB approved a *Revised Ethical and Religious Directives for Catholic Health Care Services* in 1994. This edition had six sections with several significant developments. First, it expanded beyond medical ethics to include issues of social justice. Catholic moral theology has a long-noted methodological and normative division between biomedical and sexual ethics on the one hand and social ethics on the other. Catholic social teaching formulates principles, such as the common good, for example, that allow for interpretation and application. Catholic sexual teaching and biomedical ethics often consist of absolute, one-size-fits-all norms, regardless of context and circumstances, and applicable always and everywhere, such as the prohibition of artificial contraception and direct sterilization. The 1994 *ERD* recognizes that social justice is a central consideration in health care ethics and provides a complement to, and perhaps, we will argue, a corrective for, some absolute health care and sexual norms. In his *Amoris Laetitia*, Pope Francis proposes "New Pastoral Methods" for approaching moral issues surrounding marriage and family and demonstrates an integration of Catholic social and sexual teaching that could serve as an important addition to future revised editions of the *ERD*.[12]

Second, rather than presenting a more positive approach to Catholic identity, previous editions of the *ERD* emphasized a series of negative prohibitions of what Catholic hospitals and health care professionals cannot do. The 1994 *ERD* intended to create a culture dedicated to promoting human dignity "in a way that was animated by the spirit of the Gospel and guided by the teachings of the Church." Third, it expands its treatment of clinical issues to include advance directives, reproductive technologies, and artificial nutrition and hydration and offers theological justification for its ethical conclusions. We argue that this theological justification is insufficient, given the Church's deficient anthropology and methodology to justify its teachings. Fourth, in tune with the merger of Catholic and non-Catholic facilities, this edition provides guidelines for the shifting paradigm of delivery systems. The basic question here is if, and how, Catholic hospitals maintain their Catholic mission, identity, and culture when they partner with non-Catholic providers. This challenge is exacerbated today when such partnerships are essential for the very survival of Catholic health care institutions.

Each section of the 1994 *ERD* contains an explanation of the theological foundation for the specific directives in that section. There is also an appendix explaining the principle of "cooperation in evil" that was especially relevant in a time of mergers between Catholic and non-Catholic health care institutions. The Congregation for the Doctrine of the Faith (CDF) reviewed the *ERD* before the bishops voted to adopt them, but it had not reviewed the appendix on the principle of cooperation, one of the most difficult principles in Catholic moral theology to understand and apply. The appendix is a truncated explanation of this principle, and it raised concerns about interpretation among both bishops and moral theologians. In 2000 the CDF required the NCCB to review the appendix since it was open to misinterpretation and misapplication. The appendix was dropped in the 2001 edition, and all the revisions from the 1994 edition occur in part 6, "Forming New Partnerships with Health Care Organizations and Providers."

Jesuit Kevin Wildes notes two important paradigm shifts in the 1994 directives. First, there is an ecclesiological shift, a move away from a unity-in-plurality model of the Church, already reflected in different spiritualities and ministries in the Church such as those of the Jesuits and Dominicans, to a hierarchical uniformity in which the bishop is the sole arbiter for the interpretation and application of the *ERD*. This hierarchical dimension, as we shall see, has been expanded in the 2018 edition of the *ERD* and, in complex health care mergers that cross diocesan boundaries, may pit one bishop's interpretation of the *ERD* against another's. Second, there is a methodological shift from different ethical methods for discerning complex ethical issues guided by personal conscience and prudence, teleology, casuistry, and virtue ethics, for instance, to a largely deontological, rule-based, absolutist approach that too often ignores the complexity of the issues and removes the prudential judgment of conscience from the process by deductively imposing and demanding obedience to universal rules.[13]

The *ERD* was revised again in 2001, and Kevin O'Rourke, Thomas Kopfensteiner, and Ronald Hamel note four significant changes in that edition. First, directive 70 was added, forbidding immediate material cooperation with an intrinsically evil action, such as direct sterilization. Second, a footnote on directive 70 stated that it supersedes the NCCB's 1977 commentary on the 1975 CDF document *Quaecumque Sterilizatio*. The NCCB commentary agreed with the CDF that preventive sterilizations were direct and could never be performed in Catholic hospitals, but it allowed for direct sterilizations on the basis of immediate material cooperation due to duress or fear that a Catholic hospital would close if it did not perform direct sterilizations.[14] Third, the appendix on the principle of cooperation was deleted since its different interpretations and applications caused disagreement and confusion. Fourth, the concept of scandal as it is used in the principle of cooperation is more precisely defined following the *Catechism of the Catholic Church*'s definition: "an attitude or behavior which leads another to do evil. . . . Scandal is a grave offense if by deed or omission another is deliberately led into a grave offense" (*CCC*, 2284). It is clear that scandal is a serious issue and something to be avoided, but what is not clear or defined is what constitutes scandal and how claims of scandal are to be justified. The *ERD* claims that scandal is caused when there are violations of the *ERD* due to immediate material cooperation in wrongdoings such as the distribution of contraceptives.

Scandal, however, can depend on *which* teaching of the Catholic Church is emphasized. In response to President Barack Obama's Affordable Care Act (ACA), for example, the USCCB protested against its contraceptive mandate that requires health care facilities to provide contraceptives to those who request them, arguing that such a mandate was a violation of directive 52 and might lead people to believe that Catholic health care facilities condone contraceptive practices, which cause scandal by leading others to believe that contraceptive use is morally acceptable. Others, however, focus on Catholic teaching on the authority and inviolability of a well-informed conscience, that human dignity demands the right to follow one's conscience, and that access to health care is a basic human right.[15] Scandal can be very much in the eye of the beholder, and, we ask, which claim of scandal is justified in a given situation? The assertion that an action would cause "scandal" is precisely that, an assertion, not a moral argument, and, like any assertion of right or wrong, it must be justified by sound moral argument. Given the weaknesses of the Church's arguments against contraception and the vast majority of Catholics who do not accept the argument, scandal is just as likely to be caused by the USCCB's opposition

to the ACA's contraceptive mandate as by permitting the distribution of contraceptives by Catholic health care institutions to adult patients following an
informed and responsible conscience.

The 2009 fifth edition is, for the most part, a repetition of the 1994 and
slightly revised 2001 editions, with one notable exception, directive 58. This
directive is revised in light of Pope John Paul II's address on "Life Sustaining
Treatments and Vegetative State" and addresses in detail artificial nutrition and
hydration for dying patients. We address this revised directive in detail in chapter 1.[16]

BRIEF OVERVIEW AND ANALYSIS OF THE 2018 *ERD*

The most recent 2018 sixth edition of the *ERD* is identical to the 2009 fifth
edition, with the exception of part 6 where there are substantial revisions. We
will treat those revisions in detail in chapter 6. Briefly, the revisions focus on
"collaborative arrangements" (*ERD*, 23) between Catholic and non-Catholic
institutions, the importance and explanation of the principles guiding formal
and material cooperation, the importance of avoiding "scandal" in collaborative arrangements, references to canon law, and the significance of Catholic
health care institutions as witnesses to Catholic identity as tools for assessing
collaborative arrangements. There is an emphasis on the authority of the local
bishop to interpret and apply the *ERD* and a greater emphasis on centralizing
this authority: "The ultimate responsibility for the interpretation and application of the directives rests with the diocesan Bishop" (*ERD*, 25). In a sense, this
continues the emphasis on hierarchical centralization that Wildes notes in the
1994 edition, but it ignores the communion ecclesiology mandated by the Second Vatican Council, which we deal with in chapter 4. It also seems to ignore
the cultural and economic shifts in health care delivery that exist in partnerships
that cross diocesan boundaries and that may include multiple bishops in the interpretation and application of the *ERD*. The sixth edition takes no account of
differences between bishops in their interpretation and application of the *ERD*
and of how to resolve those differences. The general structure of the edition
is as follows: a preamble, general introduction, six parts treating various topics
and issues, and a brief conclusion.

Preamble

The preamble begins by noting that health care in the United States is subject to "extraordinary change" (*ERD*, 4). Change is manifest in technological

advances; institutional and social factors that include the changing demographics of Catholic health care employees due to the declining number of religious,
social, and cultural pluralism; delivery and collaborative arrangements in health
care; and developments in Catholic moral theology since the Second Vatican
Council. All of these changes present challenges to moralists, health care personnel, and bishops who are to interpret and apply the *ERD*. Methodologically,
the preamble mentions "the aid of other sciences" (*ERD*, 4) over the centuries
to develop numerous moral principles that constitute the *ERD*; we will address
this point in detail in chapter 3. The *ERD* states two purposes: "first, to reaffirm
the ethical standards of behavior in health care that flow from the Church's
teaching about the dignity of the human person; second, to provide authoritative guidance on certain moral issues that face Catholic health care today"
(*ERD*, 4). It then lays out the structure of the *ERD*, which consists of six parts
divided into two sections. The first section is expository: "It serves as an introduction and provides the context in which concrete issues can be discussed
from the perspective of the Catholic faith." The second section is prescriptive:
"Directives promote and protect the truths of the Catholic faith as those truths
are brought to bear on concrete issues in health care" (*ERD*, 5).

General Introduction

The foundation of the *ERD* is Jesus' healing ministry testified to in the gospels (*ERD*, 6) and continued in history in the Church's compassionate health
care ministry. The introduction makes several important points on ecclesiology and methodology. First, commentaries on the revised *ERD* note a focus
on emphasizing the local bishop's authority to interpret and apply the *ERD*
and to promote collaboration among health care leaders, employees, ministers,
theologians, "approved authors," and specialists.[17] The bishop is to serve as
pastor, teacher, and priest. As pastor he promotes and encourages the faithful to
participate in the Church's healing ministry; as teacher he ensures the religious
and moral identity of health care ministries throughout the diocese; as priest
he ensures sacramental care for the sick (*ERD*, 7).

Methodologically, the *ERD* draws from the four sources of ethical knowledge, scripture, tradition, reason, and experience, to justify its principles that
facilitate protecting and attaining human dignity. It emphasizes the importance of dialogue between science and faith and the importance of a "correct
conscience based on the moral norms for proper health care" (*ERD*, 7). There
is some overlap in the introduction between the ecclesiological and methodological considerations. The bishop has the final say on how the *ERD* is to be
interpreted and applied. When an issue arises where the magisterium has not

offered a determinative answer, "the guidance of *approved authors* can offer appropriate guidance for ethical decision making" (*ERD*, 7). Conscience, which we deal with in detail in chapters 2 and 6, is mentioned without explanation only in the final sentence of the introduction. "Each person," it states, "must form a correct conscience based on the moral norms for proper health care" (*ERD*, 7). These moral norms are defined by the magisterium and interpreted by the bishop and his "approved authors." There is a clear ecclesiological and methodological hierarchy in the *ERD*. The local bishop has ultimate authority on both the authoritative interpretation and application of the *ERD* and the determination of the "approved authors" to guide him in making his authoritative judgment. The hierarchy of the four sources of ethical knowledge are established as follows: tradition, narrowly defined as magisterial teaching and the authority of the local bishop to interpret and apply those teachings; scripture as interpreted by the magisterium; reason that conforms to magisterial teaching; and experience. There is no mention of a traditional and essential source of ethical knowledge, namely, the *sensus fidelium*. Experience is mentioned twice in the entire *ERD*. The first is in reference to patients' experiencing human dignity (*ERD*, 10), and the second is in reference to the experience of health care professionals to pursue healing, to maintain health, and to provide compassionate care (*ERD*, 13).

Six Parts

The body of the *ERD* is divided into six parts, each of which includes an introduction and specific directives. Part 1, "The Social Responsibility of Catholic Health Care Services," is spelled out in five points. First, Catholic health care ministry is committed to promoting and defending human dignity, which is foundational to Catholic moral teaching and to the *ERD*. The concept of human dignity grounds a theological anthropology, which we explore in detail in chapter 2 and which is foundational for formulating and justifying specific directives that facilitate and do not frustrate human dignity. Second, there is an emphasis on the biblical mandate to care for "the poor, the uninsured and underinsured; children and the unborn; single parents; the elderly; those with incurable diseases and chemical dependencies; racial minorities; immigrants and refugees" (*ERD*, dir. 3). We could surely add the underpaid, the unemployed, and the homeless to that list. Third, Catholic health care ministry is committed to realizing the common good: "economic, political, and social conditions [that] ensure protection for the fundamental rights of all individuals and enable all to fulfill their common purpose and reach their common goals" (*ERD*, 8). Fourth, Catholic health care ministry must practice responsible stewardship and the responsible use and distribution of limited resources. Discernment of the use of resources is guided by the principle of subsidiarity or participatory justice, which includes dialogue with anyone who seeks to participate but especially those, including the most vulnerable, who are directly affected by resource distribution. Fifth, part 1 recognizes that, in a pluralist society, individuals may request medical procedures that are "contrary to the moral teachings of the Church" (*ERD*, 8) and asserts that denying those requests does not offend the individual conscience. We explore the interrelationship between the authority of magisterial teaching and the authority of individual conscience in chapter 2.

Part 2, "The Pastoral and Spiritual Responsibility of Catholic Health Care," emphasizes human dignity and that each and every person created in the image of God (Gen. 1:26) shares in that dignity. The physical dimension is central to the care and treatment of every patient, but the *ERD* emphasizes holistic care of the person physically, psychologically, socially, and spiritually: "Without health of the spirit, high technology focused strictly on the body offers limited hope for healing the whole person" (*ERD*, 10). Pastoral care is an essential component of Catholic health care and the healing process and must provide for the spiritual needs of the patient. Priests, deacons, religious, lay chaplains, and all Catholic health care personnel act in complementary ways to provide pastoral care through healing ministry. In this part, the *ERD* employs a holistic anthropology, recognizing that the person is an integrated being physically, psychologically, spiritually, and relationally. We have two preliminary comments on part 2. First, this holistic anthropology is inconsistently recognized when it comes to specific directives, especially with respect to sexual ethical issues and the beginning and end of life. Second, as Sister Jean deBlois comments, the section on pastoral and spiritual care is "woefully inadequate."[18] We address these points in chapter 1 and chapter 5, respectively.

Part 3, "The Professional-Patient Relationship," explains and promotes "a truly interpersonal professional-patient relationship" (*ERD*, 13). Health care professionals must provide professionally competent and compassionate care, informing patients about their health care issues and guiding them to maintain or restore health, taking into account the patient's convictions, values, and spiritual needs. Patients depend on health care providers to promote the holistic health of body, mind, and spirit and to restore health or preserve life. Patients are responsible for using these resources to realize holistic health in light of their spiritual and moral commitments. Patient autonomy and health care recommendations are limited in the patient-physician relationship by the Catholic identity of the institution, which trumps patient autonomy and recommended medical practice. The *ERD* summarizes the interrelationship between the patient, health care professional, and the Catholic institution: "When the health care professional and the patient use institutional Catholic health care, they also accept its public commitment to the Church's understanding of and witness to the dignity of the human person" (*ERD*, 13).

The interrelationship between patient, physician, and the identity of the Catholic institution raises several questions. First, through its directives guiding the patient-physician relationship and teachings regarding specific ethical issues, the Church posits a theological anthropology or definition of human dignity and what facilitates and does not frustrate human dignity. This theological anthropology, as we show, is not always consistent. Second, there is a question of moral agency and who has the right and authority to decide and on what criteria. At times, the patient, the health care professional, or the Catholic institution has that authority. Third, related to the question of authority, what is the relationship between the conscience of the patient, the health care provider, and the Catholic institution? Which voice should have authority, and what are the criteria for making that determination? We attempt to respond to those questions as we proceed.

Part 4, "Issues in Care for the Beginning of Life," notes that Catholic health care emphasizes the sanctity of life "from the moment of conception until death" (*ERD*, 16). It focuses on sexual intercourse in marriage and addresses two ethical issues related to it, contraception and reproductive technologies. It quotes *Gaudium et Spes* to explain the mutual self-giving and procreative meanings of conjugal love, and it quotes *Humanae Vitae* to emphasize the unitive and procreative meanings of sexual intercourse. It recognizes responsible parenthood that allows a married couple to limit the number of children "by natural means" and follows *Humanae Vitae* in prohibiting "contraceptive interventions" (*ERD*, 16). It then claims that reproductive technologies, which substitute for the marital act, violate human dignity. It summarizes: "Just as the marriage act is joined naturally to procreation, so procreation is joined to the marriage act" (*ERD*, 17). There are several points to make regarding the introduction to part 4. First, it fails to acknowledge Pope Francis's recent statements on marriage and the family that natural methods of fertility regulation are to be "promoted" (*AL*, 222). This is very different from *Humanae Vitae*'s and the *ERD*'s absolute condemnation of contraception, which is nowhere quoted in *Amoris Laetitia*. Second, Pope Francis notes that the married couple should make any decision about fertility regulation in conscience before God. Here and elsewhere Francis reinstitutes the authority and inviolability of conscience, which the *ERD* consistently fails to recognize. Third, the *ERD* employs a sexual anthropology that prioritizes the biological over the relational, psychological, and spiritual dimensions of human sexuality. The focus is entirely on the conjugal act of intercourse and its procreative meaning, not on its relational meaning. It states, with no supporting evidence aside from the Church's interpretation of natural law, that contraception and reproductive technologies are destructive of human dignity and imposes this vision on all married couples. We address the anthropological and methodological issues raised in part 4 in chapters 2 and 3, respectively.

Part 5, "Issues in Care for the Seriously Ill and Dying," begins by emphasizing Christ's redemptive and saving grace, which is present and active at all times, including when a person is facing sickness, suffering, and death. This part emphasizes the virtues of faith, hope, and humility when facing suffering and death; the virtue of prudence when making end-of-life decisions on what is ordinary and proportionate care and what is burdensome and disproportionate care; and the assurance that Catholic health care will be a community of love, support, and respect. Euthanasia and physician-assisted suicide are absolutely prohibited, but a patient may in good conscience forgo disproportionate or burdensome treatment. The *ERD* includes numerous references to the virtues, but the directives often prioritize obedience to Church teaching over every other virtue. A particularly challenging issue in part 5 is the 2009 addition of directive 58, requiring the use "in principle" of medically assisted nutrition and hydration for patients in a persistent vegetative state. The challenges for this directive, as we shall see, relate to moral agency: who decides, what are the criteria for that decision, and how is the decision made?

Part 6, "Collaborative Arrangements with Other Health Care Organizations and Providers," includes the only substantial changes from the fifth edition and is crucial to navigating the ongoing complex social, cultural, economic, and contextual dimensions of collaborative health care delivery. The introduction to this section is unique in that it explains in some detail the principles of legitimate material and formal cooperation as the foundational principles guiding collaborative relationships. These principles were first included in the appendix in the 1994 edition of the *ERD*, but that appendix was dropped in the 2001 and 2009 editions because "experience has shown that the brief articulation of the principles of cooperation that was presented there did not sufficiently forestall certain possible misinterpretations and in practice gave rise to problems in concrete applications of the principles."[19] The principles themselves are still included in the 2001 and 2009 editions (dir. 69 and 70, respectively), with a more expansive explanation of the principles in the 2018 edition. We explore the complexity of understanding, interpreting, and applying these principles in chapter 6.

We note a few important points about part 6. First, it recognizes that pursuing the common good may require collaboration with institutions "that do not operate in conformity with the Church's moral teaching" (*ERD*, 23). This is an important point in that it recognizes a hierarchy of values; the common good can be a greater good that justifies collaboration with institutions that do not follow Catholic teaching. It has long been recognized in Catholic moral theology that values can come into conflict and that there must be criteria or principles for resolving any conflict. The *ERD* often cites proportionate reason as such a principle, determining what benefits can outweigh burdens in end-of-life decisions, for example, or the principles of legitimate cooperation to address questions of collaboration. Second, "particular circumstances" can help in making this prudential judgment, and they must be taken into account. Circumstances are important since they specifically address context; prudential judgment means that reasonable people may disagree on how the principle is interpreted and applied in particular collaborative arrangements. Third, part 6 asserts without adequate explanation that scandal is to be avoided. Fourth, "reliable theological experts should be consulted" (*ERD*, 24). Fifth, the diocesan bishop is responsible for interpreting and applying the directives and for recruiting reliable experts to help him in his interpretation. This raises the question of collaborative relationships that extend beyond one diocese into another and how to resolve disagreements between bishops in a particular collaborative relationship or in interpreting and applying the *ERD*. We address the principles guiding cooperation and the ecclesiological considerations in this analysis and evaluation in chapters 6 and 4, respectively.

METAETHICS

We begin our critical analysis of the *ERD* with the most basic question of ethics. Many people understand ethics to be primarily about what is good or right, but the most fundamental question of ethics is whether the terms *good* or *right* have any meaning. If they do not, is there such a thing as ethics? Do ethical terms have meaning against which we can evaluate reality or human experience, or do they merely express sentiments, feelings, or emotions that contain no criteria for determining their truth or falsity? Until this question is answered we cannot proceed to the next question in ethics, which is the definition of ethical terms and the formulation and justification of norms for attaining the ethical good. In this section, we first explore the metaethical theory of the Catholic tradition, namely, natural law, for the *ERD* asserts that "the moral teachings that we profess here flow principally from the natural law, understood in the light of the revelation Christ has entrusted to his Church" (*ERD*, 4). Second, we propose perspectivism as a metaethical epistemology that accounts for plural definitions of the good defined as human dignity.

Ontology: Physicalist or Personalist?

The classification of ethics that attempts to answer the question of whether or not there is ethical truth, or whether the terms *good* or *right* and their opposites have any meaning, is known as *metaethics*. *Meta* derives from the Greek meaning "to go beyond" or "transcend." The area of ethics called metaethics attempts to define the very foundation of ethics. It asks the most basic questions of whether there is such a thing as ethical truth, whether ethical terms have meaning, and whether that meaning can be justified. There are two distinct areas in metaethics, ontology and epistemology.[20]

Ontology investigates the *foundation* on which ethical truth is based; epistemology investigates how we *know* ethical truth. The Catholic metaethical tradition, grounded in a physical understanding of natural law, claims that we can define the good and that we can justify that definition based on various sources of ethical knowledge. Thomas Aquinas provides the classic Catholic definition of natural law: human participation in eternal law through right reason (*ST*, I–II, 91, 2). Ontologically, natural law posits that God created both the universe and an ethical order to the universe that human beings, through reason, can know and understand. There are at least two understandings of this ontological truth in the Catholic tradition, physicalism and personalism.[21] The first understanding, and the one that predominates in Catholic sexual ethics and much of biomedical ethics, defines the ethical as physical, biological reality, commonly referred to as physicalism. Physicalism emphasizes the biological and physical dimensions of human dignity: prioritizing the biological and physical dimensions over all other dimensions is ethically right, and violating the biological and physical dimensions is ethically wrong. For example, the physical structure of the sexual act is directed toward reproduction, and to impede or disrupt this physical act, through contraception or sterilization, for example, is a violation of the natural law and is morally wrong. Reproductive-type sexual acts between a married couple are right and moral; contraceptive sexual acts between a married couple are wrong and immoral, and so are all non-reproductive sexual acts that cannot reach their biological finality.

The second understanding of ontological truth focuses on relationship and is often designated as personalism. Personalism defines human dignity in terms of what facilitates interpersonal relationship: what is right facilitates interpersonal relationship, and what is wrong frustrates it. When the focus is on relationship, the answer to the question of whether or not a contraceptive act disrupts the biological finality of the sexual act is not ethically decisive. What is decisive is the answer to the question of how this act affects one's human relationships. If a contraceptive act frustrates relationship, it is morally wrong;

if it facilitates relationship, it is morally right. The relational meaning of the act is ethically prioritized over its biological or physical meaning, and the physical act becomes a, not the, dimension of the relationship. Generally speaking, in Catholic theological ethics it is not an either/or ontology, either physicalism or personalism, but both/and. Catholic natural law ethics recognizes the morality of both the biological and the relational, but it is a question of which is to be prioritized on a specific ethical issue and situation.

Both Pope John Paul II and many traditionalist moral theologians and Pope Francis and many revisionist moral theologians, for instance, claim to be personalists; that is, they recognize the human person in relationship as a source of ontological truth. These groups have, however, very different theological anthropologies and definitions of human dignity and the moral norms that facilitate or frustrate human dignity. Pope John Paul II and traditionalist moral theologians, for instance, maintain that the use of contraceptives always frustrates human dignity and is, therefore, immoral; Pope Francis and revisionist moral theologians maintain that contraception may be either right or wrong depending on how it impacts human relationship. What accounts for this normative difference is an ontological prioritization of the relational or physical. John Paul II, in what some label a "theology of the body," prioritizes the physical dimension of human dignity as essential and determinative to fulfill the relational dimension. John Finnis, a staunch traditionalist philosopher and defender of Church teaching on human sexuality, states this prioritization explicitly: acts of a reproductive kind are "biologically *and thus* personally [or relationally] one."[22] In his human person adequately considered, revisionist moral theologian Louis Janssens prioritizes the relational dimension of human dignity as essential and determinative, the biological or physical being a, but not the, determining dimension of human dignity.[23] The ethical implications are clear. For John Paul II and traditionalist moral theologians, contraception by definition frustrates human dignity and damages the marital relationship, disrupting the physical structure of the marital act by separating its procreative and unitive meanings. For Janssens and revisionist moral theologians, contraception may or may not frustrate human dignity depending on the relational meaning of their sexual intercourse for the spouses. The ontological prioritization of the physical or relational meaning of the sexual act divides the two interpretations of natural law and their definitions of human dignity.

Epistemology: Ecclesial Positivism or Perspectivism?

The two interpretations of natural law are divided epistemologically as well. Traditionalist and revisionist theologians fundamentally disagree on how human beings *know* natural law. David Kelly argues that Church teaching represented in the *ERD* is a type of epistemological positivism. Positivism is a metaethical epistemology that claims that the definition of human dignity and the norms and principles that follow from that definition are imposed or posited without any rational or ontological basis. Ecclesial positivism maintains that the Church posits its definition of human dignity, norms, and principles without rational or ontological justification. Kelly notes that this epistemology took root in the early twentieth century, when hierarchical pronouncements on medical ethical issues gained prominence and influence both in theological literature and in Church teaching. Church authority supplemented and often replaced the scientific competence of Catholic moral theologians to discern the meaning and ethical nature of the natural law tradition.[24] Tracing the history of this shift toward ecclesiastical positivism, Kelly explores the work of the leading Catholic medical ethicist in the United States in the 1950s, Jesuit Gerald Kelly, who notes, "The Church not only claims divine authorization to interpret the moral law, it also claims that its teaching is a practical necessity for a clear and adequate knowledge of this law."[25] This authority, combined with a physicalist understanding of moral agents and their acts, promotes a legalistic, absolutist, obedience-to-rules-based morality, especially in the areas of sexual and medical ethics.

Although we agree, in part, with Kelly's assessment that Church teaching is guilty of ecclesiastical positivism and that Church authority has replaced the professional competence of Catholic moralists to discern, know, and understand natural law, its definition of human dignity, and the norms and principles that follow from that definition, we disagree with the ontological implications of positivism that there is "no rational or ontological basis" for what the Church teaches. We believe that there is a shared commitment to natural law in both official Church teaching and revisionist moral perspectives, an ontology of what is physical or biological and what is relational. The primary difference between the two perspectives is the prioritization of a physicalist or relational ontology and the definition of human dignity that flows from that prioritization. Theologian Bernard Lonergan's epistemology of perspectivism accounts for these differences. We first explain this epistemology and then the various definitions of human dignity evident in Catholic teaching and reflected in the *ERD*.

Perspectivism

Lonergan proposes perspectivism as an epistemological theory that can account for plural definitions of human dignity and of any other moral issue. According to perspectivism, different truths derive from different theoretical perspectives.

This theory reliably and adequately accounts for different definitions of human dignity and the norms that facilitate or frustrate it. It also addresses charges of relativism aimed at those who disagree with some of the absolute norms the Church teaches. Writing on the nature of historical knowledge, Lonergan states, "Where relativism has lost hope about the attainment of truth, perspectivism stresses the complexity of what the historian is writing about and, as well, the specific difference of historical from mathematical, scientific and philosophic knowledge."[26] Relativism concludes to the falsity of a judgment. Perspectivism concludes to its *partial* but reliable and adequate truth and, therefore, also to the further development of that truth toward its fullness.

Lonergan offers three factors that give rise to perspectivism in human knowledge, including moral knowledge. First, human knowers are finite, the information available to them at any given time is incomplete, and they cannot attend to or master all the data available to them. Second, the knowers are selective, given their different socializations, personal experiences, and the range of data offered to them. Third, knowers are individually different, and we can expect them to have different interpretations of the data available to them. The theologian-knower immersed in the philosophy of Plato, Saint Augustine for instance, will achieve different understanding, make different judgments, and act on different decisions from a theologian-knower immersed in the philosophy of Aristotle, Saint Thomas Aquinas for instance. Augustine and Aquinas produce legitimate but different theologies, both of which are necessarily partial and incomplete explanations of complex theological reality. They are like two viewers at fourth-story and thirteenth-story windows of the Empire State Building; each gets a different, but no less partial, reliable, and adequate view of what lies outside their windows. We could expect that if they both ascended to a higher story, they would get a different, but still no less partial, reliable, and adequate view.

Every human judgment of truth, including every judgment of moral truth, is a limited judgment based on limited data and understanding. "So far from resting on knowledge of the universe, [a judgment] is to the effect that, no matter what the rest of the universe may prove to be, at least *this* is so."[27] It is precisely the necessarily limited and, as neuroscience teaches us, sometimes inhibited nature of human sensations, understandings, judgments, and decisions that leads to perspectivism, not as to a source of falsity but as to a source of partial but reliable and adequate truth. Though he said it on the basis of his understanding of God's incomprehensibility, Augustine's restating of earlier Greek theologians is apropos and accurate here: "*Si comprehendis non est Deus*, if you understand, what you understand is not God."[28] Aquinas articulates the same judgment differently: "Now we cannot know what God is, but only what

God is not; we must, therefore, consider the ways in which God does not exist rather than the ways in which God does."[29]

No single objectivist definition of human dignity comprehensively captures its full truth. Perspectivism accounts for the plurality of partial truths embedded in different definitions. It is an epistemology that presents limited persons as they exist, that attends to those dimensions of the person deemed most important for defining human dignity, that interprets and prioritizes those dimensions if and when they conflict, and that formulates and justifies norms that facilitate, and do not frustrate, the attainment of human dignity. The only way for humans to achieve truth is via perspectives that are partial and particular.[30] Focus on and effortful attention to different particular perspectives leads to both different and partially true definitions of human dignity and the formulation of different norms that facilitate or frustrate it. Such different definitions, we will argue throughout, may be reconciled in charitable dialogue.

In summary, there is broad metaethical agreement within Catholic theological ethics. First, it accepts some version of metaethical objectivism; there *are* objective definitions of human dignity. Second, it defines the ethical terms *good* and *right* in relation to some objective definition of human dignity. Third, given different perspectives and theological lenses, Catholics can and sometimes do disagree on both the specific definition of human dignity and the formulation and justification of norms that facilitate or frustrate its attainment. Fourth, Bernard Lonergan's theory of perspectivism, which recognizes the inherent limitations of humans to know, accounts for the different definitions of human dignity and the different formulations and justifications of norms that facilitate or frustrate it. Fifth, the variability that arises from perspectivism is an essential part of an objectivism that recognizes universals; the good is *objectively* defined as human dignity. Different objective definitions of human dignity are to be taken as necessarily partial definitions, not as forms of relativism that deny universals.

TENSIONS IN THE *ERD*

In light of our historical overview and introduction to the content of the *ERD* and our introduction to metaethics, we believe that, although the *ERD* attempts to provide clear guidelines for Catholic health care, it contains some inconsistencies. These inconsistencies are anthropological, methodological, ecclesiological, and spiritual. In what follows, chapter 1 explores the sources of ethical knowledge and their selection, interpretation, prioritization, and integration to justify the good defined as human dignity and to formulate and justify norms that facilitate, and do not frustrate, attaining human dignity. Chapter 2 explores various definitions of human dignity in Church teaching and points out anthropological inconsistencies in the *ERD*. Based on Pope Francis's theological anthropology, it proposes a holistic definition of human dignity that requires substantive revisions to the existing *ERD*. Chapter 3 investigates the methodological disconnect and tension between Catholic social, sexual, environmental, and medical ethical teaching and where these tensions are evident in the *ERD*. Chapter 4 focuses on ecclesiology. It explores the ecclesiology at work in the *ERD* in relationship to the bishop, how he exercises authority in relation to Catholic health care in his own diocese, his relationship with other bishops and how conflicts between them are to be resolved, and the role and function of the *sensus fidelium* in discerning the directives. Chapter 5 focuses on pastoral ministry and spiritual care in Catholic health care and explores its strengths and weaknesses in light of contemporary religious, social, and cultural developments. Chapter 6 explores collaborative arrangements between Catholic and non-Catholic health care providers and critically analyzes the principles governing cooperation and related concepts. Chapter 7 concludes our commentary on the *ERD* with suggestions on how to revise its next edition.

SUGGESTED READINGS

Griese, Orville N. *Catholic Identity in Health Care: Principles and Practice.* Chapter 1. Braintree, MA: Pope John Center, 1987.

Kaveny, Cathleen. "Pope Francis and Catholic Healthcare Ethics." *Theological Studies* 80, no. 1 (2019): 186–201.

Kelly, David F., Gerard Magill, and Henk Ten Have. *Contemporary Catholic Health Care Ethics,* 2nd ed. Washington, DC: Georgetown University Press, 2013.

McCormick, Richard A. *Health and Medicine in the Catholic Tradition: Tradition and Transition.* New York: Crossroad, 1984.

O'Rourke, Kevin, Thomas Kopfensteiner, and Ronald Hamel. "A Brief History: A Summary of the Development of the *Ethical and Religious Directives for Catholic Health Care Services.*" *Health Progress* 82, no. 6 (2001): 18–21.

Salzman, Todd A., and Michael G. Lawler. "Natural Law and Perspectivism: A Case for Plural Definitions of Objective Morality." *Irish Theological Quarterly* 82, no. 1 (2017): 3–18.

NOTES

1. See Cathleen Kaveny, "Pope Francis and Catholic Healthcare Ethics," *Theological Studies* 80, no. 1 (2019): 186–201.

2. See David F. Kelly, *The Emergence of Roman Catholic Medical Ethics in North America: An Historical-Methodological-Biographical Study* (New York: Edwin Mellen Press, 1979). Revisions to the *ERD* were made in 1956, 1971, 1994, 2001, 2009, and 2018.

3. Richard A. McCormick, *Health and Medicine in the Catholic Tradition: Tradition and Transition* (New York: Crossroad, 1984); Orville N. Griese, *Catholic Identity in Health Care: Principles and Practice* (Braintree, MA: Pope John Center, 1987).

4. Gerald Kelly, SJ, *Medico-Moral Problems* (Saint Louis, MO: Catholic Hospital Association of the United States and Canada, 1958), vii.

5. McCormick, *Health and Medicine*, 6.

6. Ethicists of the NCBC, "An Introduction to the Sixth Edition of the ERDs," *Ethics and Medics* 44, no. 1 (January 2019): 1–4, at 1.

7. See Dennis M. Doyle, *Communion Ecclesiology* (Maryknoll, NY: Orbis, 2000); Michael G. Lawler and Thomas J. Shanahan, *Church: A Spirited Communion* (Collegeville, MN: Liturgical Press, 1995).

8. "Where the *Ethical and Religious Directives* Fall Short," *Health Progress* (May–June 2009), available at https://www.chausa.org/publications/health-progress/article/may-june-2009/where-the-ethical-and-religious-directives-fall-short.

9. We are indebted in this section to Kevin O'Rourke, Thomas Kopfensteiner, and Ronald Hamel and their article, "A Brief History: A Summary of the Development of the *Ethical and Religious Directives for Catholic Health Care Services*," *Health Progress* 82, no. 6 (2001): 18–21, for their overview of the *ERD* up to the 2001 fourth edition.

10. Kelly, *Medico-Moral Problems*.

11. It should be noted that although Pope John Paul II condemned proportionalism in *Veritatis Splendor* as an ethical method, the *ERD* in particular and Catholic teaching in general continue to use proportionate reason as an established principle in discerning responses to ethical questions. There is often a failure to distinguish between proportionalism as an ethical method and proportionate reason as an ethical principle within magisterial documents and among traditionalist theologians.

12. See Todd A. Salzman and Michael G. Lawler, "*Amoris Laetitia*: Towards a Methodological and Anthropological Integration of Catholic Social and Sexual Ethics," *Theological Studies* 79, no. 3 (2018): 634–52.

13. Kevin Wm. Wildes, SJ, "A Memo from the Central Office: The 'Ethical and Religious Directives for Catholic Health Care Services,'" *Kennedy Institute of Ethics Journal* 5, no. 2 (June 1995): 133–39. See also David F. Kelly, "Methodological and Practical Issues in the Ethical and Religious Directives for Catholic Health Care Services," *Louvain Studies* 23 (1998): 321–37.

14. See David F. Kelly, Gerard Magill, and Henk Ten Have, *Contemporary Catholic Health Care Ethics*, 2nd ed. (Washington, DC: Georgetown University Press, 2013), 284–89.

15. See *GS*, 16; *DH*, 2–3; *AL*, 37, 42, 222.

16. Pope John Paul II, "Address of John Paul II to the Participants in the International Congress on 'Life-Sustaining Treatments and Vegetative State: Scientific Advances and Ethical Dilemmas,' Saturday, 20 March 2004," available at http://w2.vatican.va/content/john-paul-ii/en/speeches/2004/march/documents/hf_jp-ii_spe_20040320_congress-fiamc.html.

17. Ethicists of the NCBC, "Introduction."

18. "Where the *Ethical and Religious Directives* Fall Short."

19. *Ethical and Religious Directives for Catholic Health Care Services*, 4th ed. (Washington, DC: USCCB, 2001), 36; *Ethical and Religious Directives for Catholic Health Care Services*, 5th ed. (Washington, DC: USCCB, 2009), 30–31.

20. See Todd A. Salzman, *Deontology and Teleology: An Investigation of the Normative Debate in Roman Catholic Moral Theology* (Leuven, Belgium: Peeters Press, 1995).

21. For a helpful explanation of these two perspectives, see Brian V. Johnstone, C.Ss.R., "From Physicalism to Personalism," *Studia Moralia* 30 (1992): 71–96.

22. John Finnis, "Law, Morality, and 'Sexual Orientation,'" *Notre Dame Law Review* 69, no. 5 (1994): 1049–76, at 1067; emphasis added.

23. Louis Janssens, "Artificial Insemination: Ethical Considerations," *Louvain Studies* 8 (1980): 3–29.

24. Kelly, *Emergence*, 364.

25. Kelly, *Medico-Moral Problems*, 31–32.

26. Bernard J. F. Lonergan, *Method in Theology* (New York: Herder, 1970), 217.

27. Bernard J. F. Lonergan, *Insight: A Study of Human Understanding* (London: Longmans, 1957), 344, emphasis added. See also Lonergan, *Method in Theology*, 217–19.

28. *Sermo* 52, 16, *PL*, 38, 360; International Theological Commission, "Theology Today: Perspectives, Principles and Criteria," November 29, 2011, 97, available at http://www.vatican.va/roman_curia/congregations/cfaith/cti_documents/rc_cti_doc_20111129_teologia-oggi_en.html. For a detailed analysis, see Victor White, *God the Unknown* (New York: Harper, 1956); and William Hill, *Knowing the Unknown God* (New York: Philosophical Library, 1971).

29. *ST*, I, 3, Preface.

30. Bryan Massingale, "Beyond Revisionism: A Younger Moralist Looks at Charles E. Curran," in *A Call to Fidelity: On the Moral Theology of Charles E. Curran*, ed. James J. Walter, Timothy O'Connell, and Thomas A. Shannon (Washington, DC: Georgetown University Press, 2002), 253–72, at 258.

CHAPTER ONE

The Sources of Ethical Knowledge and Tensions in the *ERD*

In this chapter we explore the traditional sources of ethical knowledge and how their selection, interpretation, prioritization, and integration (SIPI) lead to different perspectives on the teachings and directives of the revised *ERD*. Before we embark on our critical analysis of the *ERD*'s selection of the sources of ethical knowledge and its ethical method, however, we preface an important caveat. The *ERD*'s preamble specifies that the document has "been refined through an extensive process of consultation" that included bishops, theologians, physicians, administrators, sponsors, and other health care providers. It further specifies that the *ERD* provides "standards and guidance" but does not "cover in detail all of the complex issues that confront Catholic health care today." It commits the *ERD* to periodic review "in light of authoritative Church teaching, in order to address new insights from theological and medical research or new requirements of public policy" (*ERD*, 4). The primary objective of the *ERD* is not to be a systematic reflection on ethical method or the SIPI of ethical sources but to provide moral and pastoral guidelines for Catholic health care institutions based on Church teaching. In our critical analysis, therefore, we can only deduce the ethical method of the *ERD* and its SIPI of the sources of ethical knowledge on the basis of Church ethical teaching in general. We review the case of Bishop Thomas J. Olmsted of Phoenix to evaluate the SIPI of the Catholic sources of ethical knowledge in the *ERD* and to demonstrate why future revisions of the *ERD* ought to include additional methodological clarifications on how to interpret and apply the *ERD* when conflicts between bishops arise.

THE SOURCES OF ETHICAL KNOWLEDGE AND ETHICAL METHOD

We begin our exploration of the sources of ethical knowledge and ethical method with a definition. Theologian Bernard Lonergan defines method as "a normative pattern of recurrent and related operations yielding cumulative and progressive results."[1] Operations comprise such processes as gathering evidence, understanding, marshaling, and evaluating the evidence, making judgments, and deciding to act. To construct a normative pattern, ethical method must account for both epistemic claims about how we know ethical truth and normative claims about how we justify the content of that truth and apply it in specific cases. Catholic ethical method is a theological method that proposes both an epistemology for reaching ethical truth and a normative pattern for reaching a definition of human dignity and formulating and justifying norms for its attainment. The epistemology we follow in this work, as discussed in the introduction, is perspectivism that recognizes plural claims for the definition of human dignity. By common theological agreement, the sources of Christian ethical knowledge to construct and justify a normative ethics are found in what is known as the Wesleyan Quadrilateral, four established sources of Christian ethical knowledge, namely, scripture, tradition, science, and human experience.

More than fifty years ago the Second Vatican Council's *Gaudium et Spes* wisely instructed all people of good will to discern "the signs of the times" (*GS*, 4) and to interpret them in light of the Gospel. Although the content of this scrutiny has changed and evolved over fifty years, especially in health care ethics, the sage advice remains an ongoing invitation and challenge. Some of the tools suggested to guide us in this discernment process are "the experience of past ages, the progress of the sciences, and the treasures hidden in the various forms of human culture, by all of which the nature of [humanity] . . . is more clearly revealed and new roads to truth are opened" (*GS*, 44). Science and experience, which always includes culture, along with scripture and the Christian tradition, comprise the Wesleyan Quadrilateral.

We use the Quadrilateral to respond to the call from the Second Vatican Council for the renewal of Catholic theological ethics and to explain a Catholic ethical method in health care for the twenty-first century. We do so for five reasons. First, the Quadrilateral includes the sources of ethical knowledge we judge essential for doing Christian ethics, sources highlighted in various ways in Church teaching in general and in the documents of the Second Vatican Council in particular. Second, these four sources are essential to any *Christian* discernment of what is right or wrong, good or bad, though particular perspectives, as we shall see, select, interpret, prioritize, and integrate the sources in different ways. Third, there is a growing appreciation for and specific reference to these sources in Catholic ethical literature from divergent perspectives, though there remains the need for dialogue to investigate how the sources are to be selected, interpreted, prioritized, and integrated.[2] This dialogue will clarify the use of the sources and illuminate plural perspectives. Depending on their SIPI of the sources, different people may well reach different normative conclusions on medical ethical issues. Some will conclude that removing Terri Schiavo from artificial nutrition and hydration (ANH) was wrong; some will conclude it was right. Some will conclude direct sterilization is always wrong; some will conclude it can, on occasion, be right. Perspectivism accounts for these plural judgments.

Fourth, Christian ethics is grounded in faith in a God of love, compassion, and justice, and from this God we can derive meaning in life and find inspiration to realize a pacific resolution of conflict. The four sources of ethical knowledge, scripture, tradition, science, and experience, can guide us in our analysis, evaluation, and response to complex medical ethical issues that confront us on a daily basis and can invite a comprehensive and comprehensible response. Fifth, use of these four sources combined informs Catholic ethics to construct a normative pattern for a comprehensive, credible, and consistent ethical method to guide both the Church's teaching in health care ethics and individuals' formation of their well-formed consciences. The sources are methodological components facilitating a perspectivist and developing understanding of human dignity and of the norms that facilitate its attainment. *Gaudium et Spes* and, as we shall see in chapter 3, Pope Francis's *Amoris Laetitia* and *Laudato Si'*, provide revolutionary methodological insights that serve as "manifestos" for Catholic ethics to aid all people of good will and institutions in the search for ethical truth.[3]

THE SOURCES OF ETHICAL KNOWLEDGE

Catholic ethics draws on four sources: scripture, tradition, science, and human experience. We consider each in turn.

Scripture

The Second Vatican Council's *Decree on Priestly Formation* prescribes that the scientific exposition of moral theology "should be more thoroughly nourished by scriptural teaching" since scripture is the "very soul of sacred theology."[4] Any Catholic ethical method must integrate scripture and demonstrate how it functions in its method. When using scripture, two things must be kept in mind. First, when investigating the role of scripture in a particular ethical method, it is important to recognize that contemporary readers of scripture bring their own perspectives and presuppositions to the text. A crucial part of any investigation of Catholic ethics is to bring these perspectives and presuppositions to the fore in order to comprehend a particular method more fully.[5] Second, the attempt to incorporate scripture into an ethical method is akin to coherently integrating the full mystery of the divine reality to which scripture attests. Sacred scripture, a collection of diverse books from diverse times and cultures, seeks to reveal the mystery of God, but this mystery is so incomprehensibly rich that it can never be grasped in a single citation or perspective.[6] Saint Augustine teaches this most firmly in his theological statement, "Si comprehendis non est Deus," if you understand, it is not God you understand.[7]

The fullness of revelation, Christians believe, is not contained in a scriptural book. It is contained in a person, the person of Jesus the Christ, who even after his incarnational revelation remains a mystery. The project of developing an ethical method cannot be content with mystery, and as a result, there is a fundamental tension between the truths contained in scripture and how those truths are used in Christian ethics. Christian ethics will never contain the fullness of revelation, no more than does Christian scripture, though it can reflect certain parts of that revelation that, while no doubt important and foundational, do not tell the whole story. The use of scripture in Catholic ethics is similar to the viewers at fourth-story, thirteenth-story, and twenty-first-story windows of the Empire State Building; each gets a different but no less partial view. The richness of scripture and the mystery to which it attests defy full human comprehension, though there are methodological guidelines from magisterial documents for interpreting it.

In his encyclical *Divino Afflante Spiritu*, Pope Pius XII laid the foundation for the methodological integration of scripture into ethical method by endorsing the historical-critical method for its interpretation. This method was reaffirmed by the Second Vatican Council's *Dei Verbum*, which prescribes that scriptural texts are to be read in the "literary forms" of the writer's "time and culture."[8] The Pontifical Biblical Commission's *The Interpretation of the Bible in the Church* continues in this line, teaching that "Holy Scripture, in as much as it is 'the word of God in human language,' has been composed by human authors in all its various parts and in all the sources that lie behind them. Because of this, its proper understanding not only admits the use of [the historical-critical] method but actually requires it." The commission insists that "the scientific study of the Bible requires as exact a knowledge as possible of the social conditions distinctive of the various milieus in which the traditions recorded in the

Bible took shape."[9] An authentic Catholic approach to reading biblical texts could not be clearer: it is to be done using a historical-critical methodology.

Of particular relevance to this book is the commission's application of its principles for biblical exegesis to Catholic theological ethics. The Bible is God's word to the Church, but "this does not mean that God has given the historical conditioning of the message a value which is absolute. It is open both to interpretation and being brought up to date." It follows, therefore, that it is not sufficient for ethical judgment that the scripture "should indicate a certain moral position," the moral legitimacy of slavery or the prohibition of homosexual acts, for example, "for this position to continue to have validity." We have to undertake a process of understanding the text in its sociohistorical context and of discerning its contemporary relevance "in the light of the progress in moral understanding and sensitivity that has occurred over the years."[10] It is for these reasons that Jesuit Joseph Fuchs can assert correctly that what Augustine, Aquinas, and the Council of Trent said about ethical behavior cannot exclusively control what theological ethicists say today.[11] We must understand, judge, and apply scripture according to the "signs of the times," in dialogue with the other sources of ethical knowledge, all in a particular historical-cultural context.

Discovering what scripture says about ethics, therefore, is never as straightforward as simply reading a scriptural text. The reader must get behind the text to understand how the Church and its theologians interpret it and apply it to contemporary ethical issues. The Second Vatican Council issued instruction on how the scriptures of both Testaments are to be read:

> To search out the intention of the sacred writers, attention should be given, among other things, to "literary forms." For truth is set forth and expressed differently in texts which are variously historical, prophetic, poetic, or of other forms of discourse. The interpreter must investigate what meaning the sacred writer intended to express and actually expressed in particular circumstances by using contemporary literary forms in accordance with the situation of his own time and culture.[12]

It is never enough simply to read a scriptural text to find out what it says about contemporary Christian ethics. Only after its original sociohistorical context is clarified can the text be translated, interpreted, and applied in a contemporary context.

Tradition

The second source of ethical knowledge is tradition, and it is intrinsically related to scripture. Scripture and tradition are but one source of divine revelation,

since the New Testament is itself the tradition of the earliest Christian communities. Scripture was written in a particular time and place for a particular
people and may be said to be secondary revelation, the early Christian community's written interpretations of the primary revelation, God's self-revelation in
Jesus the Christ. The word *tradition* can mean both the act of handing on the
Church's continuing interpretation of the primary revelation in Jesus and the
theological content that is handed on. Catholics believe that content in faith,
another word with two meanings. It can mean both the act of faith, actually
believing the content of tradition, and the content that is believed. There are
fundamental truths contained in tradition, trinity and incarnation for example,
and Catholics believe them, but our understanding of these truths develops
in light of contemporary advances in history, culture, reason, knowledge, and
experience. This evolution takes place not only in dogmatic but also in ethical
truths, especially with rapid developments in health care. Under the guidance
of the Holy Spirit, tradition interprets and applies the primary revelation in
Jesus and the secondary revelation in scripture in ever new and contextually
appropriate ways.

Because the impact of tradition on theological ethics is extensive and warrants far greater treatment than we can provide here, we narrow our investigation of that impact to what Sandra Schneiders presents as three meanings
of tradition: foundational gift, content, and mode. Foundational gift is the
unfolding experience of the Church in history under the guidance of "the Holy
Spirit who is the presence of the risen Jesus making the Church the Body of
Christ."[13] All Catholic ethical methods accept tradition as foundational gift,
but some fundamentally disagree over who in the Church is gifted to discern
and interpret that gift and the criteria for determining that giftedness, often
referred to as *charism*.[14] In his 1906 encyclical *Vehementer Nos*, Pope Pius X established the Catholic approach to discern that giftedness. The Church, he taught,
"is essentially an unequal society, that is, a society comprising two categories
of persons, the pastors and the flock, those who occupy a rank in the different
degrees of the hierarchy and the multitude of the faithful." This pyramidal
structure of the Church, he went on to teach, means that only clerics of the
various ranks are gifted to interpret and teach both tradition and faith, and "the
one duty of the multitude is to allow themselves to be led and, like a docile
flock, to follow the Pastors."[15] This pyramidal structure predominated in the
Catholic Church from the eleventh century until the Second Vatican Council
in the 1960s.

Richard McCormick notes correctly, however, that even in the documents
of the council there are unresolved theological tensions, which are evident in
different passages within the same document describing who are the gifted for

discerning ethical truth.[16] *Lumen Gentium*, for instance, in one section follows the lead of Pius X, teaching that "bishops who teach in communion with the Roman Pontiff are to be revered by all as witnesses of divine and Catholic truth; the faithful, for their part, are obliged to submit to their Bishops' decision, made in the name of Christ, in matters of faith and morals, and to adhere to it with a ready and respectful allegiance of mind" (*LG*, 25). In this passage, bishops are gifted to teach in communion with the pope; the common faithful are gifted to accept and obey episcopal teaching.

In an earlier section, however, *Lumen Gentium* teaches that the entire people of God, bishops and laity alike, are gifted to discern both dogmatic and moral truth: "The whole body of the faithful who have an anointing that comes from the holy one . . . cannot err in matters of belief. This characteristic is shown in the supernatural appreciation of the faith (*sensus fidei*) of the *whole* people, when, 'from the Bishops to the last of the faithful,' they manifest a universal consent in matters of faith and morals" (*LG*, 12). This gifting of the "whole people" is further affirmed in *Gaudium et Spes* and other council documents on the nature and authority of conscience. A 2014 document from the International Theological Commission, an arm of the Congregation for the Doctrine of the Faith, teaches that *sensus fidei* is "a sort of spiritual instinct that enables the believer to judge spontaneously whether a particular teaching or practice is or is not in conformity with the gospel and with apostolic faith." That instinct enables all believers both "to recognize and endorse authentic Christian doctrine and practice and to reject what is false" and "to fulfill their prophetic calling."[17] The document repeats *Lumen Gentium*'s teaching that through this spiritual instinct "the holy People of God shares in Christ's prophetic office" and that "the body of the faithful as a whole, anointed as they are by the Holy One (cf. Jn 2:20, 27), cannot err in matters of belief."

Discerning who is gifted in the Church has implications for Schneiders's second meaning of *tradition*, namely, content. Content is "the sum total of appropriated and transmitted Christian experience, out of which Christians throughout history select the material for renewed syntheses of faith."[18] The content of tradition is drawn from scripture, early fathers of the Church, councils, and official teachings of the magisterium, the ongoing theological reflection within the Church in dialogue with culture, science, experience, and *sensus fidei*, "the instinctive capacity of the whole Church to recognize the infallibility of the Spirit's truth."[19] The content from these sources must be critically selected, understood, and interpreted for its ongoing truth and usefulness for the present moral life of the Church, using the same historical-critical method that is used for understanding and interpreting scripture. If found not useful for advancing Catholic ethical life, traditional content must be renewed, as was the traditional content related to the denial of the right to religious freedom, or it may be discarded, as was the traditional content related to slavery. The coherence of traditional content must also be debated in light of human experience, as is the case with pregnancies that endanger the life of the mother and fetus and how to address the ethical issues such cases present, one of which we address later in this chapter.

Judging who among the people of God is gifted and who has the authority to discern, interpret, and transmit the content of ethical truth are all linked to Schneiders's third meaning of *tradition*, mode. Mode is the way "content is made available to successive generations of believers, the way in which the traditioning of the faith is carried on throughout history."[20] The point is frequently made that how one understands the role of the teaching authority within the Church is intimately linked with one's ecclesiology, or how one understands the nature of Church.[21] One's ecclesiology is central to how one understands tradition as mode and the role and function of the magisterium in relation to the rest of the people of God, theologians, and faithful.

Since the Second Vatican Council, Catholic theologians have generally adhered to one of two fundamentally different ecclesiological models. The model that predominated in the second millennium is a hierarchical model, according to which the content of revelation and tradition flows downward from the magisterium to the faithful. The role and function of theologians in this model is to make clear to the faithful the teaching of the magisterium but not to question or challenge that teaching. Experience and *sensus fidei* are both sources of ethical knowledge, but the magisterium must determine how those sources are to be selected, interpreted, prioritized, and integrated into its teaching. In cases where there is a disparity between the faith of the people of God and the teaching of the magisterium, as is now the case with norms prohibiting contraception, sterilization, and reproductive technologies, the magisterium gives the definitive interpretation of the meaning of human experience for human dignity and the formulation and justification of norms that facilitate or frustrate its attainment. If we think of this hierarchical model as a pyramid, the magisterium is at the pinnacle and is the hermeneutical key for the SIPI of all sources of ethical knowledge.

The Second Vatican Council introduced a renewed model of Church and, by implication, a renewed model of ethical epistemology, namely, a people of God or communion model.[22] In this model, ethical knowledge is selected, interpreted, prioritized, and integrated through the people of God, magisterium, theologians, and faithful alike. A trialogue among these three groups is guided by the Holy Spirit, with scripture, tradition, science, and human experience at the center. It is this ongoing trialogue, always conducted in mutual charity, that moves the pilgrim Church forward in history toward a fuller knowledge, understanding, and judgment of the truth of God's self-communication to God's human creatures. The magisterium maintains authority in this model, and there is a presumption of the truth of its teaching, but its authority is qualified by its role as learner as well as teacher. The faithful in general and theologians in particular can facilitate, contribute to, and sometimes even challenge and correct non-infallible magisterial teachings in this learning-teaching process. Dominican Yves Congar points out that obedience to Church authority is required when the Church is conceived on the pyramidal, hierarchical model and dialogue and consensus are required when it is conceived on the people of God-in-communion model. He adds the historical note that "it is certain that this second conception was the one that prevailed effectively during the first thousand years of Christianity, whereas the other one dominated in the West between the eleventh-century reformation and Vatican II."[23] Certainly, Pope Francis embraces the people-of-God-in-communion model in his emphasis on dialogue and synodality.[24]

Science

The sciences aid in reflecting on, analyzing, and evaluating all forms of human experience and are essential sources of ethical knowledge to define human dignity, to formulate and justify directives that facilitate attaining human dignity, and to form consciences. Pope John Paul II states that "the Church values sociological and statistical research when it proves helpful in understanding the historical context in which pastoral action has to be developed and when it leads to a better understanding of the truth" (FC, 5) and laments the fact that theologians have not fully utilized the sciences in exploring theological questions. He also highlights the need for intense dialogue between science and theology. Theology and science must enter into a "common interactive relationship" whereby, while maintaining its own integrity, each discipline is "open to the discoveries and insights of the other."[25] Physicist Ian Barbour proposes a fourfold typology of the relationship between theology and science: conflict, independence, dialogue, and integration.[26] Particularly germane to theological ethics are dialogue and integration.

The *dialogue* typology explores parallels in method, content, and boundary questions in science and theology. It seeks out similarities and dissimilarities between the methods of each discipline that may serve and complement the methods of the others. Boundary questions delimit the capabilities of each discipline and stipulate how far each may go in explanation of reality. The *integration* typology encompasses a systematic synthesis of science and religion.

Barbour's dialogue and integration typologies parallel John Paul II's proposal for a "community of interchange" between theology and science to expand the partial perspectives of each to form a new unified vision. An important caveat, however, must be heeded: theology should not seek to become science, and science should not seek to become theology in terms of either method or content; "unity always presupposes the diversity and the integrity of its elements." Neither science nor theology should become less itself but rather more itself in a dynamic interchange. Each discipline retains its own autonomy and language yet draws knowledge and insight from the other.[27] On ethical issues such as ANH and the permanent vegetative state patient, population control and contraception, and homosexuality and same-sex parenting, ecclesial authority has not always served as a wise guide in incorporating the insights of science.[28]

Human Experience

We agree with Dominican ethicist Servais Pinckaers that human experience has "a very important function in moral theology" and with *Gaudium et Spes*'s emphasis on the relevance of that experience for theological reflection.[29] Theologically interpreted past and present human experience helps to construct a definition of human dignity and to formulate and justify norms to facilitate its attainment; experience serves as a window onto the ethically normative. To deny the ethical relevance of human experience for assisting in the definition of human dignity reflects a reductionist methodology in which the only legitimate human experience is that which conforms to and confirms established Church teaching. It was such a methodology, in large part, that allowed the magisterium's approbation of slavery until Pope Leo XIII's rejection of it in 1890 and its denial of religious freedom until the Second Vatican Council's approbation of it in 1965. John Noonan comments with respect to the magisterium's late condemnation of slavery, "It was the *experience* of unfreedom, in the gospel's light, that made the contrary shine clear."[30]

A legitimate question arises at this point: Whose experience is to be used in the definition of human dignity and in the formulation and justification of norms that facilitate its attainment? We emphasize that human experience is only one part of the Wesleyan Quadrilateral and never a stand-alone source of theological ethics. "My experience" alone is never a legitimate source. Ethical authority is granted only to "our experience," to communal experience, as a source of ethical knowledge, and only in constructive conversation with the three other sources, scripture, tradition, and science, as well as with the theological reality called *sensus fidei*, the sense of the faithful and their lived experience. We must clarify what we mean by *experience*.

There is little to be gained from simply encountering the world in which we live; many people have many such encounters and learn little from them. In the Wesleyan Quadrilateral, *experience* means "the human capacity to encounter the surrounding world consciously, to observe it, be affected by it, and to learn from it."[31] The essence of such experience is never raw, neutral encounter with the world. The essence is always encounter interpreted and socially constructed by both communities and individuals in specific sociohistorical contexts. It is, therefore, also dialectical, differently construed, perhaps, by "me," by "you," by "us," and by "them," by neo-Thomist, neo-Augustinian, and revisionist theologians, for instance. For genuine human experience as we have defined it, the dialectic is necessarily a "dialectic of reason *and* experience," never controlled by either reason or experience alone. It is also a dialectic that results not in an absolutist ethical code but in "various revisable rules."[32] In a Church that is a communion of believers, the resolution of different construals of experience to arrive at ethical truth requires a respectful, charitable, and prayerful dialogue, such as that lauded and rhetorically embraced by Pope John Paul II and Pope Francis.[33] Charitable dialogue must occur internally, among the communion of believers, some of whom are laity, some of whom are theologians, and some of whom are bishops, including the bishop of Rome, all of whom acquire knowledge through experience. Dialogue must take place also externally, among all people of good will. In the formation of Church teaching and of individual conscience, people are tasked to discern what human experience confirms or challenges their definition of human dignity and, correspondingly, to formulate and justify norms that facilitate its attainment.

THE *ERD* AND THE SOURCES OF ETHICAL KNOWLEDGE

We turn now to an examination of the selection, interpretation, prioritization, and integration of the Catholic sources of ethical knowledge in the *ERD*. The *ERD* reflects a clear hierarchy in the SIPI of the sources of ethical knowledge. It bases its understanding of human dignity, the morality of human acts, and the ends that shape those human acts in natural law, "understood in the light of the revelation Christ has entrusted to his Church" (*ERD*, 4), and it narrowly defines Church as hierarchical magisterium. If the magisterium has not given a specific answer to a medical ethical question, then "the guidance of *approved authors* can offer appropriate guidance for ethical decision making," though this can never be "contrary to Church teaching" (*ERD*, 7; emphasis added). Tradition, narrowly defined as hierarchical magisterium, is the primary source of ethical knowledge in the *ERD* and serves as the hermeneutical lens for the SIPI of the sources of ethical knowledge. The diocesan bishop, with or without consultation, has ultimate moral authority to interpret and apply the *ERD* in his diocese (*ERD*, 7).

The sources to support the *ERD*'s expository and prescriptive sections are prior Church teachings, statements, encyclicals, apostolic exhortations, the *Catechism*, and canon law. The citing of earlier Church teaching to defend the *ERD* gives weight to David Kelly's claim that "ecclesiastical positivism" is the primary epistemology in Catholic health care ethics in general and in the *ERD* in particular. The *ERD* uses Church teaching to formulate and justify its own teaching, regardless of whether there are other sources of ethical knowledge that challenge the teaching or whether specific directives are in conflict with it.

The *ERD* uses scripture in a limited way. It is referenced in the introduction to detail Christ's healing ministry and the continuation of this ministry in Catholic health care, in part 2 on the pastoral and spiritual responsibilities of Catholic health care, and in the conclusion to highlight Jesus' care for and healing of the poor. The *ERD*'s use of scripture, however, is narrowly focused and limited. For example, the introduction cites the parable of the Good Samaritan to highlight the mercy and compassion health care workers show toward patients. This is certainly an important but also narrow interpretation of the parable and leaves unaddressed other agents in health care, especially the bishop as the definitive interpreter of the *ERD*. It could be asked if he exercises authority like the parable's priest, Levite, or Samaritan. Experience, a third source of ethical knowledge, is mentioned only twice in the *ERD*, once to refer to the knowledge and experience of physicians (*ERD*, 13) and once to refer to patients who experience human dignity through Catholic health care (*ERD*, 10). There is no reference to experience as a source of ethical knowledge informing the *ERD*, which remains no more than a restatement of Church norms on controversial ethical issues. The *ERD* notes that it has been "refined through an extensive process of consultation" with bishops, theologians, physicians, and others, which implies that experience factors into this refinement, but there is no indication of how or if experience has impacted any refinement. In fact, the *ERD* clearly states that anything that challenges Church teaching must be rejected (*ERD*, 7) even, we add, if grounded in the experience of faithful Catholics. Experience in the *ERD* is unidirectional. "Authoritative Church teaching" is the basis for analyzing and evaluating all experience; experience may not challenge, inform, or revise that teaching (*ERD*, 4). On important issues of human sexuality and some absolute health care norms, human experience that affirms the Church's absolute norms is judged to be authentic human experience; human experience that does not affirm them is judged to be inauthentic experience.

The fourth source of ethical knowledge is science, and the Catholic Church has an abysmal historical record of integrating science and its conclusions into its anthropological and theological understandings of reality. One need only remember the Church's condemnation of Galileo for defending a heliocentric model of the solar system or the suspicion of science in Pope Pius IX's *Syllabus of Errors* to see how true that claim is. The *ERD* replicates this limited use of science. Directive 58, for example, mandates providing ANH "in principle" for patients in a persistent vegetative state (PVS) but declares it optional if it would cause "significant physical discomfort." It is significant that physical discomfort is the primary criterion for whether or not ANH might be optional for the PVS patient, yet another example where the ontology justifying Church teaching is grounded in the physical rather than in the personal and relational. Directive 58 is also medically, and therefore ethically, questionable. A basic medical question is whether the PVS patient can experience pain or physical discomfort. The medical answer to this question has evolved. In 2007, three years after an address by Pope John Paul II on which directive 58 is based, David Kelly, citing conclusions of the American Academy of Neurology from 1989, wrote that despite PVS patients' ability for reflex actions, such as breathing, smiling, and opening their eyes, "they are totally unconscious and cannot experience pain and suffering in any way."[34] In 2018 the Academy of Neurology issued a revised statement on PVS patients' perception of pain, which asserted that "some studies using functional imaging indicate that brain activation in networks supporting pain perception is lower in patients diagnosed with PVS compared with those in MCS [minimally conscious state], suggesting that patients in PVS lack capacity for full pain awareness." Good ethical medical practice must be guided by accurate medical science. Pope John Paul II's statement in 2004 and the USCCB's inclusion of that statement in the 2009 edition of the *ERD*, directive 58, did not reflect the current state of medical knowledge on PVS patients' ability to experience pain. The medical state of the question has continued to evolve and to indicate more tentative conclusions regarding the PVS patient's capacity to experience pain; this tentativeness should be acknowledged in both Church teaching and the *ERD*.[35]

Just as there is a limited use of human experience in some health care and sexual issues in constructing a normative pattern to define human dignity and formulate directives that facilitate attaining it, there is also a limited use of science. Too often the biological and social sciences that affirm the Church's absolute norms are judged to be good science; the sciences that do not affirm those absolute norms are judged to be bad science. One clear example of this is the CDF's statement that allowing same-sex couples to adopt children would cause "violence" to these children in that it would not be conducive to their attaining full human dignity.[36] No scientific evidence is given for this claim, and, in fact, extensive scientific evidence suggests the exact opposite: children raised in same-sex households are as healthy emotionally, psychologically, and relationally as children raised in heterosexual households. The claim of violence to children in same-sex relationships stems from Church teaching on sexual complementarity based on a strict gender binary between male and female and the scientifically unfounded ethical claim that sexual personal and relational complementarity requires this "natural complementarity" between male and female. The *ERD* is guided by this same notion of complementarity and gender binary in its directives addressing human sexuality. Science challenges claims of a strict gender binary and, therefore, the formulation and justification of norms and directives that follow from that anthropological claim.[37] We agree with Kevin Fitzgerald: in light of these scientific insights, we must revise "our understanding of sexual characteristics and gender identification and the various ways in which both can be experienced and expressed in human beings."[38] In light of contemporary scientific findings about human sexuality, sexual orientation, and gender identification, there will have to be a revision of Church norms and a formulation of new *ERD* directives.

Regarding science as a source of ethical knowledge, Church teaching ought to follow Pope John Paul II's call for an ongoing dialogue between the two, even if scientific conclusions contradict normative moral claims in Catholic teaching.[39] This ongoing dialogue needs to be applied consistently, not selectively, to all categories of ethics, sexual, social, environmental, and health care, *especially* to those categories where absolute norms prevail. Pope Francis has moved toward a greater integration of science and Church teaching, especially in *Laudato Si'*, with respect to climate change. More integration is needed, however, on health care and sexual ethical issues, such as complications with pregnancies that go beyond a cancerous uterus or ectopic pregnancy and the traditional, often physicalist, interpretation of the principle of double effect, access to contraceptives, and the care and treatment of minimally conscious state patients.

There are several points, then, to notice about the sources of ethical knowledge that guide the *ERD*. First, Church tradition, narrowly defined as the magisterium, is prioritized as the authoritative perspective for formulating, interpreting, and applying the *ERD*. Scripture, experience, and science are all dependent on that hierarchical perspective. Second, tradition as a source of ethical knowledge is limited to present Church teaching, understood by the diocesan bishop, with or without the consultation of "approved authors." Third, the *sensus fidelium* is given no consideration in the *ERD* and little or no voice in Church teaching on sexual and health care ethical issues, despite Catholic social teaching's emphasis on subsidiarity or participatory justice. Fourth, conscience, where women and men "are alone with God whose voice echoes in their depth" (*GS*, 16), is limited to obedience to Church teaching. We now illustrate the lack of an adequate method for the SIPI of the sources of ethical knowledge in the *ERD* by considering the case of Bishop Thomas J. Olmsted of Phoenix and Saint Joseph's Hospital and Medical Center (SJHMC).

BISHOP THOMAS OLMSTED AND THE SOURCES OF ETHICAL KNOWLEDGE

In November 2009 a pregnant Catholic mother of four suffering from pulmonary hypertension was admitted to Saint Joseph's Hospital with worsening symptoms. She was eleven weeks pregnant and, if her pregnancy were allowed to continue to term, her risk of death was nearly 100 percent. Her fetus also would not survive the pregnancy, with or without a medical intervention. The choice for both the mother and the medical team was either to save the mother's life or lose both lives. Judging that they were following the *ERD*, the hospital ethics committee recommended a therapeutic abortion to save the mother's life and, with the informed consent of the mother, the health care team carried out that recommendation. When Bishop Olmsted learned of the case in 2010, he accused SJHMC of violating the *ERD* by performing a direct abortion to save the life of the mother; declared Sister Margaret McBride, a member of the hospital ethics committee, "automatically excommunicated" because she consented to the procedure; and withdrew SJHMC's status as a Catholic hospital. We consider Olmsted's judgment to illustrate the sources of ethical knowledge and how they function in one bishop's interpretation and application of the *ERD*, for we believe this case clearly demonstrates that the *ERD* needs to be rewritten, with greater precision and clarification in terms of the sources of ethical knowledge.

Tradition

There are at least two relevant directives that led to conflicting ethical conclusions between Olmsted and the hospital ethics committee. The first is directive 45: "Abortion (that is, the directly intended termination of pregnancy before viability or the directly intended destruction of a viable fetus) is never permitted. Every procedure whose sole immediate effect is the termination of pregnancy before viability is an abortion." The second relevant directive is directive 47: "Operations, treatments, and medications that have as their direct purpose the cure of a proportionately serious pathological condition of a pregnant woman are permitted when they cannot be safely postponed until the unborn child is viable, even if they will result in the death of the unborn child." In his official statement declaring SJHMC no longer Catholic, Olmsted stated that the procedure was a direct abortion in "clear violation" of directive 45 since "the baby was healthy and there were no problems with the pregnancy" and "the equal dignity of mother and her baby were not both upheld."[40] The hospital ethics committee followed directive 47 in its assessment and evaluation of the case. The president of SJHMC offered the following response to Bishop Olmsted regarding the case:

> Consistent with our values of dignity and justice, if we are presented with a situation in which a pregnancy threatens a woman's life, our first priority is to save both patients. If that is not possible, we will always save the life we can save, and that is what we did in this case. . . . We continue to stand by the decision, which was made in collaboration with the patient, her family, her caregivers, and our Ethics Committee. Morally, ethically, and legally we simply cannot stand by and let someone die whose life we might be able to save.[41]

The fundamentally different responses to this case hinge on different perspectives on the SIPI of the ethical knowledge sources that informed the selection, interpretation, and application of different directives.

Second, Bishop Olmsted, following the *ERD*, consulted with Father John Ehrich, his "chief [medical] ethicist" and "approved author," to reach his decision. There were, however, other, more respected approved authors that disagreed with Olmsted's selection, interpretation, and application of the *ERD* in this case. Conservative Catholic philosophical ethicist and much "approved author," Germain Grisez, formulates an ethical argument that justifies the action of SJHMC's medical team in this case.[42] Father Martin Rhonheimer, also a much approved author, was invited by the Congregation for the Doctrine of the Faith to write and publish the book, *Vital Conflicts in Medical Ethics*. He concludes that in cases of vital conflict, cases of complicated pregnancies where the lives of both mother and child are in danger, "the decision to allow both mother *and* child to die—at least when the mother can be saved and the child will die *in any case*—is simply irrational."[43] Rhonheimer can be read as presenting an ethical argument that SJHMC was ethically justified in its decision.[44] The *ERD* seems to assume a homogenous ethical voice among approved authors. In the Olmsted affair, this was clearly not the case; there are plural perspectives on the selection, interpretation, and application of the *ERD* even among approved authors.[45] Other than an author being selected by a bishop as agreeing with Church teaching, the *ERD* establishes no criteria for the designation of "approved author."

Neither does it establish any criteria to resolve conflicts when authors disagree. Sister Carol Keehan, president of the Catholic Health Association, which operates under the auspices of the USCCB to do scholarly work on health care ethics, supported the action of SJHMC, judging that it "carefully evaluated the patient's situation and correctly applied" the ERD.[46]

Third, the vast majority of Catholic ethicists and the *sensus fidelium*, a dimension of tradition never acknowledged in the ERD or in Bishop Olmsted's responses, disagreed with his medical and ethical analysis, evaluation, and conclusion and with his actions against Sister McBride and SJHMC.[47]

Fourth, Bishop Olmsted's exclusive reliance on a narrow definition of tradition as a source of ethical knowledge, on the unquestionable authority of a diocesan bishop, and on his selection of approved authors all raise additional questions. Ecclesiologically, this hierarchical model of authority violates the Second Vatican Council's communion model of Church. As bishops consult only approved authors, those who hold a single Roman theology and function as apologists for the magisterium, other theological voices are ignored, and so too are the dialogue and synodality promoted by Pope Francis.[48] Theologians who are unapproved, those whose theologically grounded positions differ from Church teaching on non-infallible moral teaching, are discounted in the consultative process. The procedure of consulting only approved authors cuts like a two-edged sword. One edge is that a bishop may claim that a judgment on the interpretation and application of the ERD has been made with theological consultation and the agreement of theologians; the other edge is a provocation of response from theologians who have not been consulted and may disagree with an interpretation and application of the ERD. This provocation creates further polarization in an already overly polarized Church. Determining whether or not a bishop's judgment is a well-grounded analysis and evaluation of a particular directive is settled ante-factum by approved authors, leaving those excluded from the consultative process with no other option but critique post-factum. If their response is critical, as it was in the Olmsted case, they are then branded unfairly as "dissenters."

This polarized situation does not serve well bishops, theologians, the body of faithful people, or, as in this case, the patients themselves. For bishops, it creates polarization between themselves and the other two segments of the Church, the faithful people who disagree with bishops' judgments on the interpretation and application of the ERD and theologians who articulate this disagreement and formulate arguments that challenge bishops' judgments. The reflections of these two unconsulted populations in the Church are necessarily restricted to either affirming or critiquing bishops' judgments, which makes it appear that dissent among the faithful and theologians is no longer "limited and occasional" but rampant (*VS*, 4). The fact is, however, that many are forced into the inaccurate classification of dissenters because they have been deprived of a prior consultative voice that might temper both the formulation of bishops' judgments and subsequent criticism of them. Basing judgments on approved authors who hold a single Roman theology oversimplifies the complexity of many health care ethical issues that would be better clarified by open, scholarly, theological, and medical consultation. We grant that medical decisions often require a quick decision that can limit the consultative process, but ante-factum consultation and dialogue should be the norm. Such consultation and dialogue can inform bishops, theologians, faithful people, and Catholic health care institutions and help in either confirming or revising the *ERD*.

In the Olmsted case, every effort at dialogue was rejected by the bishop, as is illustrated in his one-line response to M. Therese Lysaught's twenty-three-page theological analysis and commentary on the case: "I disagree with her conclusion." Perhaps even more troubling was his response to Lloyd Dean, president of Saint Joseph's parent company, Catholic Healthcare West (CHW). Dean highlighted many competent theologians' disagreement with Olmsted's judgment that this was a direct abortion and invited him to reconsider his decision. Olmsted's response was that Dean's proposal was unacceptable since "it disregards my authority and responsibility to interpret the moral law and to teach the Catholic faith as Successor of the Apostles."[49] This response relies more on ideology, power, authority, and a hierarchical ecclesiology than on sound ethical reasoning, synodality, and a communion ecclesiology. Such an approach damages not only Olmsted's but also the magisterium's credibility at a time when it is already incredibly low as a result of the clerical sex-abuse scandal so sedulously covered up by bishops. It also undermines the scholarly discernment of faithful Catholic theologians who thoughtfully responded to the Olmsted case for the instruction of the Church in complex health care ethical issues.

Fifth, Bishop Olmsted made a judgment about both SJHMC and its parent company, Catholic Healthcare West. The former is within his diocese; the latter has health care facilities outside his diocese. What are the implications of Olmsted's decision for other health care facilities that CHW owns and operates in other dioceses? How, or does, his decision impact CHW and its standing in other dioceses and the bishops who have authority over them? CHW is based in San Francisco. When asked for comment, Archbishop George Niederauer commented that the case would initiate a dialogue with CHW's leadership on this issue but affirmed Olmsted's "authority and responsibility to interpret the moral law and to teach the Catholic faith." Interpreting the moral law and teaching the Catholic faith may differ from one diocese to another and have implications for Catholic health care that spans various dioceses, potentially resulting in what may be called "geographical morality," an issue of concern in Catholic health care ethics raised some seventy years ago. The revised *ERD* does not indicate how to resolve potential disagreements between bishops with health care systems that extend beyond a particular diocese's jurisdiction but merely indicates that bishops should "make every effort to reach a consensus" (*ERD*, dir. 69). We take up the ecclesiological and canonical challenges of how to resolve disagreements between bishops in chapter 4.

Sixth, the USCCB Committee on Doctrine's statement defending Bishop Olmsted's decision and restating Catholic teaching on the distinction between a direct and indirect abortion is unhelpful because it does not address the case's complex medical, contextual, and relational issues. It fails to mention that the fetus would have died regardless of the woman's decision to have or not have the procedure or that she had a husband and four other children.[50] The USCCB's statement missed an opportunity to move the tradition forward in making nuanced statements that address the complex medical situation of maternal pulmonary hypertension and to formulate a new directive to address the situation in light of scholarly discussion. Instead, the statement merely affirmed Olmsted's pre–Vatican II ecclesiology and restated Catholic teaching that has been applied in other medical procedures, removing the cancerous uterus of a pregnant woman, for instance, but did not address this unique medical case.

The *ERD*'s prioritization of tradition, narrowly defined as Church teaching, and of the absolute authority of a diocesan bishop to interpret and apply the directives of the *ERD*, is not warranted in light of the preferred communion ecclesiology of the Second Vatican Council. Given its failure to recognize conflicts in Church teachings, disagreements among approved authors on that teaching, and a bishop's personal selection, interpretation, and application of a particular directive that is widely disputed even by approved authors, it is highly problematic and limited in its ability to serve as a useful resource in addressing the complexity of moral issues in Catholic health care. A revised *ERD* requires acknowledgment of these conflicts and clear objective criteria for resolving them. Without those criteria, the *ERD* and the authority given to bishops to interpret and apply it raise serious questions of credibility, accountability, and transparency in health care decisions that often have a profound impact on the lives of patients, health care professionals, Catholic health care systems, and society at large.

Scripture

The approach to scripture, a common Christian source of ethical knowledge, has interesting insights to offer regarding the Olmsted affair. The great Swiss theologian Karl Barth once said that Christians should read the newspaper alongside scripture. Reading the newspaper on the Olmsted affair in light of the parable of the Good Samaritan, cited in the *ERD* (6) and applied to Catholic health care workers who should care compassionately for patients and one another, sheds light on the narrowly focused use of scripture in both the *ERD* and the Olmsted affair. The professional health ethics committee of Saint Joseph's Hospital recommended a therapeutic termination of pregnancy to save the mother's life, and the health care team carried out that recommendation. Bishop Olmsted accused Saint Joseph's of performing a direct abortion to save the life of a mother and withdrew its status as a Catholic hospital. In the parable of the Good Samaritan, one focus is on the compassion of the Samaritan, the hated outsider, who responded to the needs of the victim, in contrast to the priest and Levite, representatives of the religious institution, who pass by the victim. Who, we ask, is the victim in the Olmsted affair? The bishop himself focused on the fetus as the victim, even though it was medically clear that the fetus would die no matter what. Saint Joseph's focused on the mother as the victim, since ultimately only she could be saved. Theologian John Donahue summarizes the meaning of the parable: "The outsider provides the model of love of neighbor."[51] We leave it to the discerning reader of scripture and newspaper to make a judgment of which action represents the outsider and which action represents the insider in the Olmsted affair.

Science

When the pregnant woman was admitted to Saint Joseph's on November 3, 2009, medical tests revealed that she had "very severe pulmonary arterial hypertension with profoundly reduced cardiac output." A physician confirmed "'severe, life-threatening pulmonary hypertension,' 'right heart failure' and 'cardiogenic shock.'" The medical chart noted that the woman was informed that if her pregnancy were allowed to continue, her risk of death was "near 100 percent." The chart also notes that "surgery is absolutely contraindicated."[52] Because the fetus was only at the eleven-week stage, it could not survive outside the mother's womb but would die regardless. These medical facts are not in dispute.

Ethical medical decisions and practices must be grounded in sound science. In order to make a correct ethical judgment in any case, one must have as clear and accurate a medical diagnosis as is scientifically possible. Bishop Olmsted claims that "the baby was healthy and there were no problems with the pregnancy."[53] The *National Catholic Bioethics Center* (NCBC), which supported Olmsted's judgment that this was a case of direct abortion, asserted that "there was no evidence of any pathology of the reproductive organs, nor of the fetus, its placenta or its members." Based on the NCBC's analysis of the medical data, since there was no pathology related to the pregnancy or fetus that would warrant a therapeutic intervention, the ethical conclusion is that termination of the pregnancy was a direct abortion and violated directive 45 of the *ERD*. Olmsted's and the NCBC's medical claims strike us as scientifically reductionist since they focus only on the pregnancy and ignore the overall health situation of the fetus and the mother. Lysaught is correct to point out why this move is biologically and scientifically problematic: "Pulmonary hypertension is . . . 'located' in the lungs; but insofar as the lungs are critical for the oxygenation of the blood, which is critically important for the entire physiological organism and insofar as immediate effects of this pathology are cardiac impairment. . . . It is difficult to accept an argument which attempts to simply localize pathology."[54] Traditional arguments for indirect abortions, a cancerous uterus or an ectopic pregnancy, clearly identify the pathological organ as the uterus or fallopian tube. Even though pulmonary hypertension is not localized in the uterus in the sense that Olmsted and the NCBC require to justify an indirect abortion, the medical fact remains that the overall pathology threatened the lives of both mother and fetus. The fetus would die regardless, and if no medical intervention were performed, the mother would die as well. It is medically reductionist, therefore, to claim that "there were no problems with the pregnancy."

A sound ethical argument that takes into consideration a comprehensive perspective on the medical facts dictates a clear response to this tragic case: save the only life that can be saved. The fact that Bishop Olmsted, the NCBC, and other Catholic ethicists arrived at a very different conclusion and that the USCCB Committee on Doctrine defended Olmsted's conclusion points to a reductionist view of the medical science, a disregard for an evaluation of the overall medical situation, and the problem of a physicalist interpretation of the principle of double effect to analyze and evaluate the situation.[55] Given the science and all the other variables in the case, there seems to be a problematic pattern justifying the selection, interpretation, and application of a particular directive based on the SIPI of the sources of ethical knowledge. This problem warrants a fundamental reevaluation of both how science is used in the *ERD* and the competency of some bishops, even after suitable consultation, to digest the science and make a responsible decision in light of it.

Experience

Experience, the fourth source of ethical knowledge, raises questions with respect to its role and function in formulating and justifying Church teaching in general and *ERD* directives in particular. The surgery on the patient at Saint

Joseph's happened in late 2009; Olmsted's response was delivered late in 2010. What became evident as the disagreement between Olmsted and SJHMC unfolded is that at least two *ERD* directives apply to the case and could be selected, interpreted, and applied differently depending on the bishop's perspective and his choice of approved authors. Debating which directive should have been applied in this situation, though crucially important, is not our focus here. Our focus is the Olmsted affair. The experience of the pregnant patient and her family, the medical staff, the hospital ethics committee, the bishop, and his advisers in 2009–10 does not seem to have been considered when revising the 2018 edition of the *ERD*, with the possible exception of reemphasizing the bishop's authority to interpret and apply the *ERD*. There is no indication that this case had any impact on the recognition of the possibility of conflicts in interpreting and applying the *ERD*, resolving such conflicts, or formulating new directives in light of such conflicts.

The extensive ethical writings that accompanied the case are not merely hypothetical reflections addressing an ethical issue that earlier ethical treatises were ill equipped to address. They were written to address the lived experience of pregnant women and medical complications that arise during pregnancy, the development of medical procedures and technology, and the ethical issues these raise. The absence in the revised *ERD* of any complex medical case, of the issues it raises with respect to interpretation and application of the *ERD*, and the need for either revised or additional directives to address such cases highlights the need for the magisterium to learn from experience as a source of ethical knowledge and to incorporate it into its directives. The *ERD*'s preamble does commit to reviewing the *ERD* periodically "in light of authoritative church teaching, in order to address new insights from theological and medical research or new requirements of public policy" (*ERD*, 4). The research by Rhonheimer and other approved authors, and that also of non-approved authors, on ethical issues that arise in health care warrant review by the USCCB with a view to possible revisions of the *ERD* that include specific directives in light of the research.

SUGGESTED READING

John Paul II. "The Relationship of Science and Theology: A Letter to Jesuit Father George Coyne." *Origins* 18, no. 23 (November 17, 1988): 375–78.

Lysaught, M. Therese. "Moral Analysis of a Procedure at Phoenix Hospital." *Origins* 40, no. 33 (January 2011): 537–48.

Pinckaers, Servais. *The Sources of Christian Ethics.* Washington, DC: Catholic University of America Press, 1995.

Pontifical Biblical Commission. "Interpretation of the Bible in the Church." *Origins* (January 6, 1994): 498–524.

Rhonheimer, Martin. *Vital Conflicts in Medical Ethics: A Virtue Approach to Craniotomy and Tubal Pregnancies.* Edited by William F. Murphy Jr. Washington, DC: Catholic University of America Press, 2009.

Salzman, Todd A., and Michael G. Lawler. "Experience and Moral Theology: Reflections on *Humanae Vitae* Forty Years Later." *INTAMS Review* 14 (2008): 156–69.

Schneiders, Sandra. *The Revelatory Text: Interpreting the New Testament as Sacred Scripture.* San Francisco: Harper, 1991.

Thiel, John E. *Senses of Tradition: Continuity and Development in the Catholic Faith.* Oxford: Oxford University Press, 2000.

NOTES

1. Bernard J. F. Lonergan, *Method in Theology* (repr., Toronto: University of Toronto, 2003), 4.

2. Charles E. Curran, ed., *The Catholic Moral Tradition Today: A Synthesis* (Washington, DC: Georgetown University Press, 1999); Todd A. Salzman, *What Are They Saying about Roman Catholic Ethical Method?* (New York: Paulist Press, 2003); Tobias Winright, ed., *T&T Clark Handbook to Christian Ethics* (New York: T & T Clark, 2021).

3. See Joseph A. Selling, "*Gaudium et Spes*: A Manifesto for Contemporary Moral Theology," in *Vatican II and Its Legacy*, ed. Mathijs Lamberigts and Leo Kenis (Leuven: Peters Press, 2002), 145–62.

4. *Dei Verbum*, 24.

5. See William C. Spohn, *Go and Do Likewise: Jesus and Ethics* (New York: Continuum, 2007).

6. See Karl Rahner, *Foundations of Christian Faith: Introduction to the Idea of Christianity* (New York: Seabury, 1978), 44–81.

7. *Sermo 32, PL* 38, 360.

8. *Dei Verbum*, 12; Pius XII, *Divino Afflante Spiritu* 35 (1943): 297–325.

9. Pontifical Biblical Commission, "Interpretation of the Bible in the Church," *Origins* (January 6, 1994): 498–524, at 500, 506.

10. Pontifical Biblical Commission, 519.

11. Joseph Fuchs, *Moral Demands and Personal Obligations* (Washington, DC: Georgetown University Press, 1993), 36.

12. *Dei Verbum*, 12.

13. Sandra Schneiders, *The Revelatory Text: Interpreting the New Testament as Sacred Scripture* (San Francisco: Harper, 1991; Collegeville, MN: Liturgical Press, 1999), 72.

14. See Todd A. Salzman and Michael G. Lawler, "Theologians and the Magisterium: A Proposal for a Complementarity of Charisms through Dialogue," *Horizons* 36 (2009): 7–31.

15. Pope Pius X, *Vehementer Nos* (On the French Law of Separation) (Vatican City: Libreria Editrice Vaticana, 1906), 8.

16. Richard A. McCormick, *Critical Calling: Reflections on Moral Dilemmas since Vatican II* (Washington, DC: Georgetown University Press, 1999), 103.

17. International Theological Commission, "Sensus Fidei in the Life of the Church (2014)," 49, 2, available at www.vatican.va/roman_curia/congregations/cfaith/cti_docu ments/rc_cti_20140610_sensus-fidei_en.html.

18. Schneiders, *Revelatory Text*, 72.

19. John E. Thiel, *Senses of Tradition: Continuity and Development in the Catholic Faith* (Oxford: Oxford University Press, 2000), 47.

20. Schneiders, *Revelatory Text*, 72.

21. See, for example, Richard A. McCormick, "Some Early Reactions to *Veritatis Splendor*," in *John Paul II and Moral Theology: Readings in Moral Theology, No. 10*, ed. Charles Curran and Richard McCormick (New York: Paulist Press, 1998), 5–34, at 28–30.

22. See J. M. R. Tillard, *Church of Churches: The Ecclesiology of Church as Communion* (Collegeville, MN: Liturgical Press, 1992).

23. Yves Congar, "Reception as an Ecclesiological Reality," in *Election and Consensus in the Church*, ed. Giuseppe Alberigo and Anton Weiler, *Concilium* 77 (1962): 43–68, at 62.

24. See Pope Francis, "Address of His Holiness Pope Francis for the Conclusion of the Third Extraordinary General Assembly of the Synod of Bishops, (October 18, 2014)," available at https://w2.vatican.va/content/francesco/en/speeches/2014/october/docu ments/papa-francesco_20141018_conclusione-sinodo-dei-vescovi.html.

25. John Paul II, "The Relationship of Science and Theology: A Letter to Jesuit Father George Coyne," *Origins* 18, no. 23 (November 17, 1988): 375–78.

26. Ian G. Barbour, *Nature, Human Nature, and God* (Minneapolis: Fortress Press, 2002), 1–2.

27. John Paul II, "Relationship of Science and Theology," 377.

28. For ANH and the permanent vegetative state patient, see Kevin O'Rourke, "Reflections on the Papal Allocution concerning Care for Persistent Vegetative State Patients," *Christian Bioethics* 12 (2006): 83–97, at 92. For population control and contraception, see Todd A. Salzman and Michael G. Lawler, "Experience and Moral Theology: Reflections on *Humanae Vitae* Forty Years Later," *INTAMS Review* 14 (2008): 156–69, at 160–62. For homosexuality and same-sex parenting, compare the CDF's "Considerations regarding Proposals to Give Legal Recognition to Unions between Homosexual Persons (July 31, 2003)," 7, available at http://www.vatican.va/roman_curia/congregations/cfaith/documents/rc_co n_cfaith_doc_20030731_homosexual-unions_en.html; and Paige Averett, B. Nalavany, and S. Ryan, "Does Sexual Orientation Matter? A Matched Comparison of Adoption Samples," *Adoption Quarterly* 12 (2009): 129–51.

29. Servais Pinckaers, *The Sources of Christian Ethics* (Washington, DC: Catholic University of America Press, 1995), 91.

30. John T. Noonan, "Development in Moral Doctrine," *Theological Studies* 54, no. 4 (1993): 662–77, at 674–75.

31. Neil Brown, "Experience and Development in Catholic Moral Theology," *Pacifica* 14 (2001): 295–312, at 300.

32. Edward Collins Vacek, "Catholic 'Natural Law' and Reproductive Ethics," *Journal of Medicine and Philosophy* 17, no. 3 (1992): 329–346, at 342–43.

33. John Paul II, *Ut Unum Sint* (May 25, 1995), 28–39, available at http://www.vatican.va /content/john-paul-ii/en/encyclicals/documents/hf_jp-ii_enc_25051995_ut-unum-sint .html. See Salzman and Lawler, "Theologians and the Magisterium," 7–31; *EG*; and "Address of His Holiness Pope Francis: Conferral of the Charlemagne Prize (Friday, 6 May 2016)," available at http://w2.vatican.va/content/francesco/en/speeches/2016/may/doc uments/papa-francesco_20160506_premio-carlo-magno.html.

34. American Academy of Neurology, "Position of the American Academy of Neurology on Certain Aspects of the Care and Management of the Persistent Vegetative State Patient," *Neurology* 39, no. 1 (January 1989): 125–26; David F. Kelly, *Medical Care at the End of Life: A Catholic Perspective* (Washington, DC: Georgetown University Press, 2006), 92.

35. American Academy of Neurology, "Practice Guideline Update: Disorders of Consciousness," July 3, 2018, available at https://www.aan.com/Guidelines/Home/GetGuide lineContent/931.

36. CDF, "Considerations Regarding Proposals to Give Legal Recognition," 7.

37. See Katherine A. O'Hanlon, Jennifer C. Gordon, and Mackenzie W. Sullivan, "Biological Origins of Sexual Orientation and Gender Identity: Impact on Health," *Gynecologic Oncology* 149, no. 1 (2018): 33–42, at 40.

38. Kevin Fitzgerald, "Viewing the Transgender Issue from the Catholic and Personalized Health Care Perspective," *Health Care Ethics USA* 24, no. 2 (2016): 7–10, at 8.

39. Pope John Paul II, "Relationship of Science and Theology."

40. Bishop Thomas J. Olmsted, "St. Joseph's Hospital No Longer Catholic: Statement of Bishop Thomas J. Olmsted," *National Catholic Reporter*, December 21, 2010, http:// ncrnews.org/documents/olmsted_statement_dec21_2010.pdf.

41. St. Joseph's Hospital and Medical Center, "St. Joseph's Resolved in Saving Mother's Life, Confident Following Bishop's Announcement," *National Catholic Reporter*, December 21, 2010, http://ncrnews.org/documents/hospital_statement_dec21_2010.pdf.

42. Germain Grisez, *The Way of the Lord Jesus*, vol. 2, *Living a Christian Life* (Quincy, IL: Franciscan Press, 1993), 502–3.

43. Martin Rhonheimer, *Vital Conflicts in Medical Ethics: A Virtue Approach to Craniotomy and Tubal Pregnancies*, ed. William F. Murphy Jr. (Washington, DC: Catholic University of America Press), 123; emphasis in original.

44. Martin Rhonheimer, "Vital Conflicts, Direct Killing, and Justice: A Response to Rev. Benedict Guevin and Other Critics," *National Catholic Bioethics Quarterly* 11, no. 3 (2011): 519–40. For a commentary on Rhonheimer and Grisez and the St. Joseph's case, see M. Therese Lysaught, "Moral Analysis of a Procedure at Phoenix Hospital," *Origins* 40, no. 33 (January 2011): 537–48, available at http://epublications.marquette.edu/cgi/viewcon tent.cgi?article=1372&context=theo_fac.

45. For approved authors who agree with Bishop Olmsted's interpretation and application of the ERD, see Thomas A. Cavanaugh, "Double Effect Reasoning, Craniotomy, and Vital Conflicts: A Case of Contemporary Catholic Casuistry," *National Catholic Bioethics*

Quarterly 11, no. 3 (2011): 453–63; and Nicanor Pier Giorgio Austriaco, "Abortion in the Case of Pulmonary Arterial Hypertension: A Test Case for Two Rival Theories of Human Action," *National Catholic Bioethics Quarterly* 11, no. 3 (2011): 503–18. For approved authors who do not or would not agree with Olmsted's interpretation and application, see Rhonheimer, *Vital Conflicts in Medical Ethics*; Rhonheimer, "Vital Conflicts, Direct Killing, and Justice"; Grisez, *Way of the Lord Jesus*, 502–3; and Benedict M. Ashley, Jean K. deBlois, and Kevin D. O'Rourke, *Health Care Ethics: A Theological Analysis*, 5th ed. (Washington, DC: Georgetown University Press, 2006), 82.

46. See Jerry Filteau, "Catholic Health Association Backs Phoenix Hospital," *National Catholic Reporter*, December 22, 2010, available at https://www.ncronline.org/news/catholic-health-association-backs-phoenix-hospital.

47. See Kevin O'Rourke, "From Intuition to Moral Principle: Examining the Phoenix Case in Light of Church Tradition," *America*, November 15, 2010, available at https://www.americamagazine.org/issue/755/article/intuition-moral-principle.

48. Pope Francis, "Address of His Holiness Pope Francis."

49. Bishop Olmsted, "Letter to Dean H. Lloyd, President of CHW, November 22, 2010," available at https://www.aclu.org/files/assets/2010-11-22-bishopletter1.pdf.

50. USCCB Committee on Doctrine, *The Distinction between Direct Abortion and Legitimate Medical Procedures* (Washington, DC: USCCB, June 23, 2010), available at http://www.usccb.org/about/doctrine/publications/upload/direct-abortion-statement2010-06-23.pdf.

51. John R. Donahue, "Companions on a Journey: The Bible and Catholic Social Teaching," in *Scripture and Social Justice: Catholic and Ecumenical Essays*, ed. Anathea E. Portier-Young and Gregory E. Sterling (Lexington Books / Fortress Academic, 2018), 9.

52. Lysaught, "Moral Analysis," 538.

53. Olmsted, "St. Joseph's Hospital No Longer Catholic."

54. Lysaught, "Moral Analysis," 546.

55. See Rhonheimer, "Vital Conflicts, Direct Killing, and Justice."

CHAPTER TWO

Anthropological Tensions in the *ERD*

As noted in the introduction, we believe that Church teaching is rooted in its understanding of natural law, posits a universal definition of human dignity, and recognizes a rational and ontological basis for that definition that can be known through human reason. We are also convinced that there are inconsistent definitions of human dignity in Catholic teaching in general and in the *ERD* in particular; some directives prioritize the relational over the physical, and some prioritize the physical over the relational. In what follows we explain and critically analyze three definitions of human dignity evident in Catholic teaching, then demonstrate tensions with those definitions in the *ERD* itself.

THE *ERD* ON HUMAN DIGNITY

The *ERD* considers human dignity a foundational concept that guides the direction and tone of the document and informs its directives: "Catholic health care ministry is rooted in a commitment to promote and defend human dignity" (*ERD*, 8). Though the *ERD* does not provide a comprehensive definition of human dignity, it does note that human beings are created in the image and likeness of God (7), links human dignity to the common good (dir. 9), emphasizes the sanctity of life from conception, and upholds the dignity of marriage and the marital act of spousal intercourse (16). The preamble specifically notes that a goal of the *ERD* is "to reaffirm the ethical standards of behavior in health care that flow from the Church's teaching about the dignity of the human person" (4). Consequently, we must look to that teaching to discover how human dignity is defined.

CHURCH TEACHING ON HUMAN DIGNITY

The good in Church teaching can be defined as human dignity, human fulfill-ment, human flourishing, or some similar cognate, but there are various per-spectives that define human dignity differently depending on the specific area of Church teaching. There is not a single definition of human dignity in that teaching. We will present various definitions of human dignity that are reflected in Church teaching and consider those different definitions in light of the *ERD*. We divide these different definitions into Catholic sexual human dignity, Cath-olic social human dignity, and Catholic holistic human dignity.

Catholic Sexual Human Dignity: Complementarity

Pope John Paul II has developed the most comprehensive definition of Catholic sexual human dignity in light of both past Church teachings, notably Pope Paul VI's encyclical *Humanae Vitae* and its prohibition of the use of artificial contra-ception in every act of sexual intercourse, and contemporary ethical issues, such as reproductive technologies and the social and cultural move to recognize the morality and legality of same-sex relationships. His introduction of ontolog-ical complementarity, which includes the biological and relational dimensions of human dignity, is a foundational concept in contemporary Church teaching that defines Catholic sexual human dignity and defends the Church's absolute norms in sexual ethics.

John Paul attempted to move the Catholic tradition beyond a procreationist, physicalist ontology and develop the unitive, relational ontology of human sexuality by more fully developing personalist insights into human relationality. Sexuality, he argues, "by means of which man and woman give themselves to one another through the acts which are proper and exclusive to spouses is by no means something purely biological, but concerns the innermost being of the human person as such." This is said to be a sign of "a total personal self-giving" (*FC*, 11). John Paul develops his philosophical personalism in conjunction with a reading of scripture to construct a theological anthropology, which others have called a theology of the body. This theology is grounded in a theolog-ical anthropology, developed from Genesis, of the communion between man and woman. Masculinity and femininity are "two 'incarnations' of the same metaphysical solitude before God and the world." These two ways of "'being a body' . . . complete each other" and are "two complementary ways of being conscious of the meaning of the body." It is through the complementarity of female and male that a "communion of persons" can exist and that the two "become one flesh."[1]

Complementarity has become a foundational concept in both John Paul II's theological anthropology and Church teaching on human sexuality. Complementarity intends that certain realities belong together and together produce a whole that neither can produce alone. We note the following characteristics of complementarity. First, complementarity is nearly always classified along masculine and feminine lines.[2] Second, complementarity is often formulated as a "nuptial hermeneutics" in terms of bridegroom and bride.[3] Third, in his theological anthropology, John Paul II posits an "ontological complementarity" whereby men and women, though fundamentally equal and complete in themselves, are incomplete as a couple.[4] Sexual complementarity completes the couple in marriage and reproductive-type sexual acts by bringing the masculine and feminine biological and psychological elements together in a unified whole. All non-reproductive-type sexual acts, such as contraceptive and homosexual acts, damage this complementarity and frustrate human dignity.

All three characteristics of complementarity—male/female, nuptial, and ontological—are evident in John Paul II and Church teaching on sexual anthropological complementarity and serve as a foundation for various types of complementarity with subcategories within each type. First, in *Familiaris Consortio* John Paul discusses "natural complementarity," lauding what we refer to as biological and personal complementarity that creates "an ever richer union with each other on all levels—of the body, of the character, of the heart, of the intelligence and will, of the soul—revealing in this way to the Church and to the world the new communion of love, given by the grace of Christ" (*FC*, 19). We note three important points in John Paul's explanation of "natural complementarity."

First, there is an intrinsic relationship between biological and personal complementarity, between body and person (heart, intelligence, will, soul). Second, biological complementarity can be divided into heterogenital complementarity and reproductive complementarity. Heterogenital complementarity is the physically functioning female and male sexual organs. Reproductive complementarity is the physically functioning female and male sexual organs used in sexual acts to biologically reproduce. Heterogenital and reproductive complementarities, however, are to be carefully distinguished, for while John Paul maintains that a couple must complement each other heterogenitally, the Church also teaches that, "for serious reasons and observing moral precepts," it is not necessary that they biologically reproduce.[5] Infertile couples and couples who choose for serious reasons not to reproduce can still enter into a valid marital and sacramental relationship. While reproductive complementarity always entails heterogenital complementarity, heterogenital complementarity does not always entail reproductive complementarity. Heterogenital complementarity is distinct from and can stand alone from reproductive complementarity in the service of personal complementarity. Third, given that John Paul's theology of the body and Church teaching explicitly forbid homosexual acts, it is clear that both regard heterogenital complementarity as a sine qua non for personal complementarity in sexual acts. Without heterogenital complementarity, "natural complementarity" in the sexual act is not possible.

John Paul also discusses "ontological complementarity," which the CDF calls "affective complementarity."[6] This type of complementarity is at the crux of John Paul's teaching on the theology of the body and the sexual human person because it intrinsically links biological and personal complementarity between woman and man. John Paul claims that "even though man and woman are made for each other, this does not mean that God created them incomplete."[7] Each individual has the potential to be complete by integrating the biological, psychological, social, and spiritual elements of affective complementarity. When considering the couple, even though woman and man are "complete" in themselves, John Paul argues that "for forming a couple they are incomplete."[8] He further notes that "woman complements man, just as man complements woman. . . . Womanhood expresses the 'human' as much as manhood does, but in a different and complementary way."[9] We may reasonably ask, however, where incompleteness and the need for complementarity are to be found in an individual that is complete in herself or himself but is incomplete for forming a couple. Where in the human person is this incompleteness that needs complementing by the opposite sex found?

John Paul responds that "womanhood and manhood are complementary not only from the physical and psychological points of view, but also from the ontological. It is only through the duality of the 'masculine' and the 'feminine' that the 'human' finds full realization."[10] The masculine and feminine complement each other to create a "unity of the two," a "psychophysical completion," not only in sexual acts but also in marital life.[11] For John Paul, then, sexual intercourse between spouses is a language of the body in truth, which includes two dimensions. The first dimension pertains to the two intrinsic meanings of the sexual act, the unitive and the procreative meanings. To eliminate or suppress either meaning of the sexual act, whether in the case of contraception or reproductive technologies, falsifies "the inner truth of conjugal love."[12] The second and more fundamental dimension pertains to an anthropology based on "the nature of the subjects themselves who are performing the act."[13] Complementarity is a principle that explains this anthropology whereby, in marriage and the sexual act, the masculine and feminine biological, psychological, and spiritual elements are ontologically linked in a unified whole. These two dimensions by definition eliminate the possibility of ethical homosexual acts and ethical non-reproductive heterosexual acts, even between a married couple.

John Paul II's Sexual Anthropology: A Critique

John Paul II's personalist anthropology and Church teaching based on it are good examples of how paradigm shifts can change terminology, human nature vis-à-vis human person, and still fall prey to neo-scholastic conceptual and terminological baggage. While John Paul's works are laden with references to the person, personal dignity, and responsibility, these are frequently explained and defined in terms of "nature" and more often than not ignore the lived, relational experience of married couples.[14] He notes that "in the order of love a man can remain true to the person only in so far as he is true to nature. If he does violence to 'nature' he also 'violates' the person by making it an object of enjoyment rather than an object of love."[15] Contraception is a violent act toward "nature" and has a "damaging effect on love."[16] Love and procreation are intrinsically linked in John Paul's theology of the body and Church teaching on complementarity, but in this relationship there is a clear hierarchy of the physical over the personal and relational.[17] This prioritization is clear in John Paul's discussion of complementarity. Heterogenital complementarity is the sine qua non and primary consideration for whether or not personal complementarity can be realized. If heterogenital complementarity is not present, as it is not present in homosexual acts, the sexual act is by definition "intrinsically disordered" (CCC, 2357), and there can be no personal complementarity in it regardless of the *relational meaning* of those acts for the two persons involved.

In a personalist-based theology, however, one must ask whether or not the biological and physical can serve as an adequate foundation for the personal and relational. John Paul II and Church teaching cite Genesis 1:27 to defend the prioritization of biology in its anthropology: "Christian anthropology has its roots in the narrative of human origins that appears in the Book of Genesis, where we read that 'God created man in his own image [...] male and female he created them.'" "These words," it continues, "capture not only the essence of the story of creation but also that of the life-giving relationship between men and women, which brings them into intimate union with God."[18] Biblical scholar Athalya Brenner confirms that semantically Genesis 1–3 emphasizes a biological and, therefore, relational binary of maleness and femaleness, but that is not the contemporary Catholic understanding.[19] The Second Vatican Council abandoned the focus on *sexed bodies* and replaced it with a focus on *related persons*. In marriage, a man and a woman enter into a personal covenant in which "the spouses mutually bestow and accept each other" (*GS*, 48), not each other's bodies, as was stated in the 1917 Code of Canon Law.[20] This focus on interpersonal covenant brings marriage and all friendship relationships into line with the rich biblical traditions of covenant between God and God's people and Christ and Christ's Church.[21] John Paul II's and Church teaching's prioritization of biology over personal relationship in their use of scripture and tradition to construct their anthropology is theologically outdated. Personal, covenantal relationship between God and humanity, not biology, is dominant in scripture. All people, female and male and intersex, can enter into such covenantal relationships, each imaging the infinite God in their own unique way.

Creation's form and shape flow from God's relationship to it; they do not preexist that relationship. Relationship is primary; creation's materiality flows from that divine relationship. Even in God's creation of 'adam, humankind, "God created [hu]mankind ['adam] in his image" (Gen. 1:27). God creates humanity through relationship first, and biological, sexed bodies are a manifestation of that relational creation. John's Gospel affirms this relational prioritization. It begins with the relationship between God creator and God savior. "In the beginning was the Word, and the Word was with God, and the Word was God. . . . All things came to be through him, and without him nothing came to be" (John 1:1–4). The masculine pronoun is used to designate God as spiritual, relational being, not male-sexed, relational being. The relationship between God and Word is at the root of all creation, including the creation of female and male, which first flows from and manifests that relationship and only then reflects it in biological materiality. Humanity's shape and form derive from God's relationship with humanity. Just as Jesus' relationship with God the creator was established before Jesus' sexed humanity, so too humans' relationship with God is established before their sexed humanity as female and male. Relationship is primary; biology is secondary. In a wonderful way the reality of intersex people, though statistically a minority, confirms and privileges this relationality. It disrupts the biological heterogenital complementarity that is foundational for Catholic sexual human dignity and the absolute norms that follow from that definition.

We ask: Should not personalism begin with a holistic understanding of human people in all their psychological, emotional, relational, spiritual, and biological complexity? If this is so, then the biological is only one dimension of the person, and it should not be given inordinate importance in the hierarchy of being or as a foundation for sexual anthropology. Authentic personalism takes the particular human person in her or his sexual complexity and formulates normative guidelines for sexual relationships out of a profound appreciation of that complexity, not on the primacy of heterogenital complementarity. John

Paul II's and the Church's notion of complementarity lacks an appreciation and integration of the whole human person, biologically, psychologically, relationally, and spiritually. To the extent that the *ERD* and its directives are based on Catholic sexual human dignity in addressing sexual ethical issues such as contraceptives (*ERD*, 16 and dir. 52) and reproductive technologies (*ERD*, 17 and dir. 38, 39, 41), it also lacks this appreciation and integration of the whole person. Interestingly, directive 40, on heterologous reproductive technologies, shifts its emphasis from the prioritization of the biological, procreative meaning of the sexual act to the covenantal, relational union between the spouses. This reveals another tension in the anthropology reflected in Church teaching and in the *ERD* and introduces a distinct anthropology that prioritizes a relational ontology over a biological/physical ontology.[22]

Catholic Social Human Dignity

The definition of Catholic sexual human dignity is foundational for the *ERD*, guiding Catholic health care institutions on both sexual ethical issues and end-of-life issues such as medically assisted nutrition and hydration that "in principle" should be provided to all patients who need them (*ERD*, 20, dir. 58). It is not, however, the only definition of human dignity reflected in Church teaching or the *ERD*. Part 1 of the *ERD*, "The Social Responsibility of Catholic Health Care," couples human dignity with the Catholic social principle of the common good and introduces a distinct definition of human dignity grounded in Catholic social teaching. Citing the USCCB's document *Economic Justice for All*, the *ERD* notes, "The common good is realized when economic, political, and social conditions ensure protection for the fundamental rights of all individuals and enable all to fulfill their common purpose and reach their common goals" (*ERD*, 8). Catholic social teaching is founded on two basic principles: human dignity and the social nature of human persons.[23] We will focus on *Gaudium et Spes*'s and *Amoris Laetitia*'s definition of human dignity under Pope Francis's Catholic holistic human dignity since there is significant overlap between it and Catholic social human dignity. Catholic social human dignity is quite distinct from Catholic sexual human dignity in its emphasis on the principle of the common good as an essential anthropological dimension.

The social nature of human persons consists of recognizing the interrelationship and finding a balance between human dignity and the unique person created in the image and likeness of God and the social, political, economic, institutional, and environmental relationships in which that person exists. John Coleman labels the anthropological core of Catholic social teaching "communitarian liberalism," which consists of several interrelated dimensions: human dignity, the common good, solidarity, a preferential option for the poor, distributive justice, subsidiarity or participatory justice, and stewardship.[24] As noted, human dignity is defined differently in Catholic teaching depending on the specific ethical issue. Catholic sexual human dignity prioritizes a physical ontology over a relational ontology; Catholic social human dignity considers the complex social relational and biological dimensions of the human person and, depending on the ethical issue, may prioritize one dimension over another. For example, adequate food, clean water, and health care are essential to maintaining physical health, which takes priority over purely economic considerations and justifies governmental and nongovernmental safety nets, including funding access to health care for the poor.

A fundamental epistemological question is whether there is a single definition or plural definitions of the common good. Plural definitions would allow for plural responses to specific ethical questions. The common good and therefore Catholic social human dignity recognizes pluralism. The CDF's International Theological Commission (ITC) asserts that "in the context of pluralism, which is ours, one is more and more aware that one cannot elaborate a morality based on the natural law without including a reflection on the [subjective] interior dispositions or virtues [or perspectives] that render the moralist capable of elaborating an adequate norm of action."[25] This process of elaboration is evolving and pluralist: "The vision of the common good evolves with the societies themselves, according to conceptions of the person, justice, and the role of public power" (85). Pope Francis approvingly cites the International Theological Commission's document: "Natural law could not be presented as an already established set of rules that impose themselves *a priori* on the moral subject; rather, it is a source of objective inspiration for the deeply personal process of making decisions" (*AL*, 305). Brian Stiltner accurately notes that "pluralism is central to the common good because different communities center on the pursuit of different components [or perspectives] of the complex human good; because institutional diversity facilitates extensive participation in social life; and because no one association [including the Church and its non-infallible moral teachings] can claim to be a perfect community."[26] The challenge for the ongoing discernment of the meanings of the common good is to engage in what David Hollenbach calls "social solidarity across cultures" in order to "attain a greater degree of shared moral vision."[27] This process takes time, patience, and a commitment to the "dialogue in charity" that Popes John Paul II and Francis promote.

Just as perspectivism and Church teaching recognize plural definitions of human dignity, so too do they recognize plural definitions of the common good. The *ERD* is inconsistent in its definition of the common good. It assumes a narrow definition of the common good when it teaches absolute norms on sexual ethical issues and some end-of-life issues and a broad definition when it teaches more flexible norms on care for the poor and on end-of-life issues.

The *ERD* assumes a narrow definition of the common good when it juxtaposes the teaching authority of the Catholic Church and conscience. It states, "within a pluralistic society, Catholic health care services will encounter requests for medical procedures contrary to the moral teachings of the Church. Catholic health care does not offend the rights of individual conscience by refusing to provide or permit medical procedures that are judged morally wrong by the teaching authority of the Church" (*ERD*, 8). Such issues include sexual ethical issues and absolute norms that prohibit contraception or direct sterilization and end-of-life issues such as physician-assisted suicide. The authority of the Church parses here to the local bishop's interpretation of absolute, though non-infallible, ethical teaching in the *ERD*. In these cases, the institutional dimension of the common good supersedes conscience and human dignity. An essential dimension of the common good, human dignity requires the authority and inviolability of conscience as central to that dignity (*GS*, 16; *DH*, 3). This prioritization of Church teaching, the institution, and absolute norms over conscience contradicts the long-established tradition on the authority and inviolability of a well-informed conscience and is, therefore, a violation of human dignity and the common good. It reflects a vision of the individual conscience put forth in Pope John Paul II's *Veritatis Splendor*, which is in tension with the vision of conscience in *Gaudium et Spes* and *Dignitatis Humanae*, detailed in chapter 6.[28] A narrow definition of the common good is also evident when the *ERD* promotes stronger centralization of the bishop's authority (*ERD*, 25, dir. 69) in interpreting and applying the *ERD* and limiting consultative voices for the bishop to "approved authors" who "can offer appropriate guidance for ethical decision making" (*ERD*, 7). The emphasis on the authority of the local bishop and the limited participation in discernment and decision-making granted to others violate subsidiarity dimensions of the common good.

The *ERD* seems to embrace a broader definition of the common good when it treats of care and concern for the poor and decisions to forgo extraordinary means of preserving life due to "excessive expense" for the family or society (dir. 57). This broader definition allows for plural analyses and ethical judgments about how a decision impacts physical dimensions of the human person as well as personal, social, and economic relationships. There is a clear tension in the *ERD* between Catholic social human dignity that posits broad and pluralist definitions of the common good based on the discernment of conscience in community and Catholic sexual human dignity that posits a narrow and single definition of the common good as interpreted by the diocesan bishop and his approved authors.

Solidarity, and the conversion necessary to realize it, is a second dimension of Catholic social human dignity. Solidarity is at the heart of the theological foundations of Catholic social human dignity, and Pope Francis calls for "authentic solidarity" in social relationships.[29] He notes elsewhere that "the suffering of others is a call to conversion, since their need reminds me of the uncertainty of my own life and my dependence on God and my brothers and sisters."[30] He proposes that solidarity is a virtue that fundamentally challenges and transforms indifference to the poor and is at the heart of the Gospel and Catholic social teaching. Pope John Paul II provides a concise definition of the virtue of solidarity: "It is a firm and persevering determination to commit oneself to the common good; that is to say to the good of all and of each individual, because we are all really responsible for all" (SRS, 38). He further explains that solidarity is undoubtedly a Christian virtue. Indeed, "many points of contact between solidarity and charity, which is the distinguishing mark of Christ's disciples (cf. Jn 13:35)," can be identified.

> In the light of faith, solidarity seeks to go beyond itself, to take on the specifically Christian dimension of total gratuity, forgiveness and reconciliation. One's neighbor is then not only a human being with his or her own rights and a fundamental equality with everyone else, but becomes the living image of God the Father, redeemed by the blood of Jesus Christ and placed under the permanent action of the Holy Spirit. One's neighbor must therefore be loved, even if an enemy, with the same love with which the Lord loves him or her; and for that person's sake one must be ready for sacrifice, even the ultimate one: to lay down one's life for the brethren (cf. 1 Jn 3:16). (SRS, 48)

There are several dimensions to John Paul's understanding of solidarity as a virtue.[31] First, it recognizes the interdependence of humanity. All humans exist in some economic, cultural, political, and religious system that affects and shapes human relationships for good or ill. Second, recognizing and naming this interdependence invites a "correlative response" in solidarity; indifference is not an option. Third, the virtue of solidarity transforms interpersonal relationships within a country, culture, or institution. Those in positions of power have a moral obligation to ensure the dignity and well-being of all their people; those who are weak or poor must reject apathetic and destructive attitudes and behaviors; those in between the powerful and weak must respect the rights and dignity of all (*SRS*, 39). Solidarity goes hand in hand with a preferential option for the poor and distributive justice.

The biblical God, and the Christ whom God sent to reveal Godself, is a God of love and justice and in real historical time stands preferentially on the side of the poor and oppressed to whom God and Christ are never indifferent. All who would be truly Christian and "perfect as your heavenly Father is perfect" (Matt. 5:48) must preferentially do the same in the face of poverty and massive economic disparities between rich and poor. This "ethical imperative" of Christian discipleship is central to the Gospel and beyond debate (*LS*, 158).

The Catholic Church is almost by definition a church of the poor; Francis—both the saint and the pope—insist that it is a poor church. Since his election, Pope Francis has consistently pointed out in both word and deed the scandal of indifference and debilitating poverty in a world of plenty and the obligation of those who have riches to share with, and to create structures that ensure participation and access for, those who have not. "The right to have a share of earthly goods sufficient for oneself and one's family belongs to everyone," and "all are obliged to come to the relief of the poor, and to do so not merely out of their superfluous goods" (*GS*, 69).[32] Pope Francis echoes that declaration. "In the present condition of global society," he writes, "where injustices abound and growing numbers of people are deprived of basic human rights [such as access to health care] and considered expendable, the principle of the common good immediately becomes, logically and inevitably, a summons to solidarity and a preferential option for the poorest of our brothers and sisters" (*LS*, 158). Though it does not use the terms, the *ERD* emphasizes solidarity, an option for the poor, and distributive justice by advocating for health care as a basic right "for the proper development of life," especially for the poor, uninsured, and underinsured (*ERD*, 8 and 23, dir. 3).

Subsidiarity or participatory justice is another essential anthropological component of the common good and Catholic social human dignity. The changing demographics of laity, theologians, and clerics within the Catholic Church in general and health care institutions in particular make it even more critical to engage in dialogue at all levels to discern the formulation, interpretation, and application of the *ERD*. A more educated laity demands that the charism of teacher-learner, so central to Catholic tradition, be discerned and perhaps redefined by laity, theologians, and bishops in dialogue. That charism demands a balance between presenting new ideas that address the contextual needs, concerns, and questions of the faithful in health care and not causing scandal to the weaker among them. As clerical vocations continue to decline, and lay people continue to be more educated and active in the Church, Church governance should reflect these changes. The principle of subsidiarity in Church governance and Catholic health care institutional decision-making demands the discernment of the charism of leadership not only in clerics but also in educated laity and theologians. The exclusion of competent laity and theologians who are not "approved authors" violates the principle of subsidiarity and silences voices that ought to be heard in the process of ongoing dialogue.

Related to the principle of subsidiarity is the process of consultation by Church leaders *before* making authoritative Church pronouncements. Pope Francis has provided a model for this consultation in the processes of the synods on marriage and the family. The word *synod* is instructive; it derives from two Greek words, *syn*, which means "together," and *hodos*, which means "journey." A synod, therefore, is a journeying together, a Church synod a journeying together of all the members of the Church, laity and clerics together, toward doctrinal and moral truth. At its fall meeting of 2019, the German Bishops Conference voted to establish what it called "the synodal way," to be inaugurated on the first day of Advent in 2020, with a meeting comprising the Bishops Conference and Germany's largest lay organization, Zentalkomitee der Deutschen Katholiken. It is a very good start in a Church that is essentially a communion of believers. Pope Francis has himself modeled commitment to a synodal way of dialogue. Dialogue, he teaches, "is born from an attitude of respect for the other person, from a conviction that the other person has something good to say. It assumes that there is room in the heart for the person's point of view, opinion, and proposal. To dialogue entails a cordial reception, not a prior condemnation. In order to dialogue, it is necessary to know how to lower the defenses, open the doors of the house, and offer human warmth."[33] Dialogue, including dialogue about Catholic health care issues, should embrace not only a bishop's court theologians or "approved authors" (*ERD*, 7) but all the competent members of the Church, clerics, theologians, and laity, both those who agree and disagree with Church teaching on specific ethical issues.

Bishops must learn to appreciate theological diversity and to consider its contributions as a manifestation of the Spirit at work in the Church, not as a threat to be silenced or excluded from the table of discernment. Although the introduction of ideas that challenge official teaching may cause tension, that is no more than a way for a pilgrim Church to move toward a fuller possession of the truth about the infinite God it believes in and what the Spirit of God may be asking of it in a plural world. Pope Francis offers an example of this journey toward truth, through dialogue, in his statement on Catholic and Orthodox relations: "I am comforted to know that Catholics and Orthodox share the same concept of dialogue . . . based on deeper reflection on the one truth that Christ has given His Church and that we do not cease to understand ever better, moved by the Holy Spirit." "We must not be afraid," he continues, "of meeting and of true dialogue. It does not distance us from the truth, rather, through an exchange of gifts, it leads us, under the guidance of the Spirit of Truth, to the whole Truth (cf. John 16:13)."[34]

It is time, indeed in this time of the scandal of clerical sexual abuse it is past time, for the Catholic Church to abandon its bunker mentality of only the authority of bishops and "approved authors," which the revised *ERD* reflects, and to replace it with Pope Francis's synodality and dialogue in Catholic health care issues. Synodality reflects the ecclesiology of the Second Vatican Council that focuses on journeying together and listening to input from all quarters of the Church, laity and clerics alike, and it advocates charitable, honest, and constructive dialogue to discern God's will and the path the Catholic Church must follow to live according to that will. This requires what both John Paul II and Francis frequently refer to as "dialogue in charity." The two synods that laid the foundation for Pope Francis's *Amoris Laetitia* modeled this dialogue in a way that previous synods have not. Synodality is a central dimension of Pope Francis's papacy and will open the door, we hope, to further dialogue and development in Church ethical teaching, including teaching about health care ethics. Dialogue, of course, is not itself the endpoint. The endpoint is the truth into which the Spirit of God is guiding the Church.

Stewardship, the responsible use and allocation of limited resources, has a predominant and necessary place in the *ERD* (7, 8, 23, dir. 4, 6, 10): "The responsible stewardship of health care resources can be accomplished best in dialogue with people from all levels of society, in accordance with the principle of subsidiarity and with respect for the moral principles that guide institutions and persons" (*ERD*, 8). Importantly, the *ERD* links the principles of stewardship and subsidiarity. Discerning the responsible use and distribution of resources requires dialogue, where all people affected by stewardship decisions, especially the poor and most vulnerable, have a voice in the dialogue. The *ERD* emphasizes the importance of social and moral principles to guide persons and institutions in this dialogue. It also emphasizes "responsible collaboration" with non-Catholic institutions. In chapter 6 we consider in detail the issue of collaboration and principles of legitimate cooperation.

In summary, the *ERD* vacillates on its definition of Catholic social human dignity and the common good in relation to human dignity. A narrow definition of the common good emphasizes adherence to absolute norms in the *ERD* interpreted and applied by the diocesan bishop and his approved authors. Following these absolute norms, it is suggested, realizes the common good and facilitates attaining human dignity; violating these absolute norms violates the common good and frustrates attaining human dignity. Conscience is subservient to absolute norms and the diocesan bishop's authority. A broad definition of the common good recognizes and embraces pluralism and its impact on the definition of human dignity. It prioritizes the authority and inviolability of a well-formed conscience to analyze an ethical situation and to interpret and apply relevant norms to make an ethical judgment of conscience. This process may or may not coincide with the *ERD* and its directives. In a broad understanding of the common good and Catholic social human dignity, differences are respected and engaged through the process of dialogue. In a narrow understanding, differences are suppressed by institution and authority. Pope Francis provides a road map for resolving the tension between a narrow and broad definition of the common good and its anthropological implications for human dignity by integrating the best of Catholic sexual and social human dignity in what we label Catholic holistic human dignity.

CATHOLIC HOLISTIC HUMAN DIGNITY

In his apostolic exhortation *Amoris Laetitia*, Pope Francis has demonstrated an integration and expansion of Catholic sexual and social human dignity, and we label this integrated anthropology Catholic holistic human dignity. *Amoris Laetitia* recognizes the impact poverty has on relationships and ethical decisions. Francis offers the example of a couple who cohabit "primarily because celebrating a marriage is considered too expensive in the social circumstances. As a result, material poverty drives people into *de facto* unions" (*AL*, 294). He does not focus on these unions as a violation of the absolute norm prohibiting fornication but recognizes that socioeconomic realities profoundly impact human relationships and human decisions. This real impact is often overlooked in Church teaching that proposes one-size-fits-all norms in its prioritization of the physical over the relational in Catholic sexual human dignity. Francis focuses on relationship and the need to offer cohabiting couples a constructive response seeking to transform the social, economic, and relational challenges they face into opportunities that can lead to the full reality of marriage and family in conformity with the Gospel. These couples, he teaches, "need to be welcomed and guided patiently and discreetly" (*AL*, 294). The integration of Catholic social and sexual teaching marks a profound shift in Catholic theological ethics, leading Cardinal Christof Schönborn of Vienna to judge that *Amoris Laetitia* "is the great text of theological ethics we have been waiting for since the days of the [Second Vatican] Council."[35] Cardinal Pietro Parolin notes that it indicates a "paradigm shift" that calls for a "new spirit, a new [method]" to help "incarnate the Gospel in the family."[36] The conservative-leaning USCCB in its most recent edition of the *ERD* has not demonstrated an awareness, or inclusion, of this paradigm shift. We now present Pope Francis's Catholic holistic human dignity and compare the ethical implications of this anthropology with Catholic sexual human dignity as reflected in the *ERD* and the use of contraceptives within the marital relationship.

Pope Francis's *Amoris Laetitia* is in continuity with anthropological developments in both Catholic social and Catholic sexual human dignity and expands on those developments by emphasizing conscience, discernment, and the virtues. It also more thoroughly integrates the methods of Catholic social and sexual teaching. These developments indicate the need for the revision of some moral norms that we address in chapter 3. *Amoris Laetitia* reflects a holistic anthropology that draws from the relational emphasis in Catholic social human dignity and a relationally focused personalist anthropology in Catholic sexual human dignity. It closely reflects, in fact, the dimensions of the human person that moral theologian Louis Janssens developed nearly forty years ago in his exegesis of *Gaudium et Spes* and its preparatory document, Schema 13.[37] In *Amoris Laetitia*, the human person is a free subject, not an object (33, 153); in corporeality; the physical and spiritual are integrated (151); in relationship to the material world (277), to others (187–98), to social groups (222), and to self (32); created in the image and likeness of God (10); a historical being (193); fundamentally unique but equal to all other persons (54). There are, however, fundamental sexual anthropological developments in *Amoris Laetitia*. In its absolute proscriptive norms, Catholic sexual human dignity prioritizes the biological function of the sexual act over its relational meanings; Francis emphasizes the relational and spiritual in ethical decision-making, and this is especially evident in his emphasis on personal conscience, discernment, and virtue.

Pope Francis on Conscience

In both his encyclical *Evangelii Gaudium* and *Amoris Laetitia*, Pope Francis again brings to the fore the Catholic doctrine on the authority and inviolability of personal conscience, especially as it relates to "irregular situations" in marital and sexual relationships. Although he clearly rejects relativism and affirms objective norms (*EG*, 64), he warns that "realities are more important than ideas" and that there must be an ongoing dialectic between reality and ideas "lest ideas become detached from realities, . . . objectives more ideal than real, [and] . . . ethical systems bereft of kindness" (*EG*, 231). Sociological surveys repeatedly affirm the significant disconnect between the proscriptive norms of Church teaching on sexual ethics, the absolute norms that prohibit artificial contraception and homosexual acts, for example, and the perspectives of the Catholic faithful. According to these surveys, the majority of educated Catholics judge that these norms are detached from reality and follow their well-informed consciences to make practical judgments on these and other moral matters.[38]

Francis calls for "harmonious objectivity" where ideas "are at the service of communication, understanding, and praxis" (EG, 232). Such objectivity can be found in personal conscience, even in the consciences of atheists. In his exchange with an Italian journalist on the issue of atheists, Francis commented, "The question for those who do not believe in God is to abide by their own conscience. There is sin, also for those who have no faith, in going against one's conscience. Listening to it and abiding by it means making up one's mind about what is good and evil."[39] The "making up one's mind," we argue, is not an endorsement of relativism, which Francis clearly rejects, but an affirmation of the discernment of moral truth by conscience informed by external, objective norms and other sources like scripture, tradition, science, and experience. His early statement on conscience seems to affirm our assessment:

> We also must learn to listen more to our conscience. Be careful, however: this does not mean we ought to follow our ego, do whatever interests us, whatever suits us, whatever pleases us. That is not conscience. Conscience is the interior space in which we can listen to and hear the truth, the good, the voice of God. It is the inner place of our relationship with Him, who speaks to our heart and helps us to discern, to understand the path we ought to take, and once the decision is made to move forward, to remain faithful.[40]

This statement reflects a model of conscience very different from Francis's predecessors John Paul II and Benedict XVI.

Mary Elsbernd demonstrates Pope John Paul's reinterpretation of the traditional understanding of conscience by comparing what is said of conscience in the Second Vatican Council's Gaudium et Spes 16 and John Paul's encyclical Veritatis Splendor 53–64. Virtually every sentence from Gaudium et Spes 16 is contained in this section of Veritatis Splendor, with the exception of these sentences: "In a wonderful manner conscience reveals that law which is fulfilled by love of God and neighbor. In fidelity to conscience, Christians are joined with the rest of men in the search for truth, and for the genuine solution to the numerous problems which arise in the life of individuals from social relationships" (GS, 16). Rather than emphasizing the general and foundational principle of love of God and neighbor and the subsidiary search for truth, John Paul emphasizes "the immutability of the natural law itself," "universal and permanent moral norms" (VS, 53), "divine law, the universal and objective norm of morality," "natural law," and "commandments" (*VS*, 60). John Paul recontextualizes *Gaudium et Spes*'s "objective norms of morality" that are grounded in the dignity of the human person and that function as a "guide" to "persons and groups" in the ongoing search for responses to contemporary problems, and he proposes instead universal, unchangeable, and objective law.[41]

This is very different from Pope Francis's discussion of rules and conscience in *Amoris Laetitia*. Francis has a distinct yet traditional perspective on natural law and its norms or rules. Natural law, he writes, "could not be presented as an already established set of rules that impose themselves *a priori* on the moral subject; rather, it is a source of objective inspiration for the deeply personal process of making decisions" (*AL*, 305). He warns against reducing a moral evaluation of a person's actions on the basis of whether or not they fulfill a law "because that is not enough to discern and ensure full fidelity to God in the concrete life of a human being" (*AL*, 304). In our judgment, Pope Francis puts rules and laws in their proper place in the process of conscience formation and discernment. They are not immutable guidelines to be followed blindly but objective inspirations to a life of discipleship that fulfills the great commandments, love of God, neighbor, and self.

In *Amoris Laetitia* Francis brings to the ethical forefront the ancient, though in the recent Catholic past largely ignored, Catholic teaching on the authority and inviolability of personal conscience. His teaching on conscience is, in our judgment, one of the central teachings in *Amoris Laetitia*.[42] He judges that "individual conscience needs to be better incorporated into the Church's praxis in certain situations which do not objectively embody our understanding of marriage" (*AL*, 303) or indeed of any ethical issue. He quotes Aquinas frequently throughout the document, especially his teaching that the more we descend into the details of situations, the more general principles are found to fail (*AL*, 304; *ST*, I–II, q. 94, art. 4). The devil is always in the details. Francis concurs with Paul VI's earlier statements on Catholic social human dignity (OA, 4, 49, 50) that there is such an "immense variety of concrete situations" that his document, indeed any ethical document, cannot "provide a new set of rules, canonical in nature and applicable to all cases" (*AL*, 300). The pathway to the moral solution of any and every moral issue is the pathway not of uninformed obedience to some external rule but of an "internal forum," well-formed conscience decision, an assiduous process of discernment guided by a spiritual adviser and a final practical judgment that commands a free subject to do this or not to do that (*AL*, 300–305). Only such an informed conscience can make a moral judgment about the details of any and every particular situation. "Truth," *Dignitatis Humanae* teaches, "cannot impose itself except by virtue of its own truth, as it makes its entrance into the mind at once quietly and with power" (*DH*, 1).

Such truth, we add, is reached only after a serious and conscientious process of discernment.

We believe Pope Francis's interpretation and contextualization of conscience in relation to principles, norms, and natural law is in clear continuity with the Catholic tradition, whereas Pope John Paul's stance on conscience in relation to principles, norms, and natural law, as formulated and expressed in *Veritatis Splendor*, is in discontinuity with that tradition. The revised *ERD*, in its stance on conscience and adherence to absolute proscriptive norms in sexual ethics, follows more closely John Paul's than Francis's perspective. Francis's model appears to us more faithful to the long-established Catholic tradition and its teaching on the inviolability of conscience, which we deal with in some detail in chapter 6.

Amoris Laetitia on Discernment

The place of discernment in moral decision-making complements the role and authority of conscience and seeks to inform and form it. The emphasis on discernment in *Amoris Laetitia* is a distinct anthropological contribution to both Catholic social and sexual human dignity. Although it is hardly surprising to find discernment used frequently by a son of Ignatius of Loyola, it is surprising to find it used so centrally as a basis for guiding responsible decisions in the realm of sexual ethics. There are parallel historical developments in the reinstatement of the authority of conscience and discernment in the ethical life. Conscience was displaced in the nineteenth and twentieth centuries by magisterial authority, rules, and the demand for submission to them, as Pius X's *Vehementer Nos* clearly shows. "The Church," Pius asserted, "is essentially an unequal society, that is, a society comprising two categories of persons, the Pastors and the flock." These two categories are so hierarchically arranged that "with the pastoral body *only* rests the necessary right and authority for promoting the end of the society and directing all its members towards that end." The only duty of the flock and the flock's consciences "is to allow themselves to be led, and, like a docile flock, to follow the Pastors."[43]

This displacement of conscience was itself displaced and the primacy of conscience reinstated to its traditional centrality in Catholic ethical life first by the Second Vatican Council and now by Pope Francis. He has also reinstated the complementarity of discernment and morality. The intrinsic link between the spiritual and ethical life, so central in Aquinas and the medieval tradition, was effectively severed at the Council of Trent, where moral theology was aligned with canon law rather than with spirituality.[44] This troubling disconnection and reconnection was codified and reinforced by the manuals of moral theology that grew out of the *Ratio Studiorum*, the Jesuit model of study, which controlled the education of seminarians up to the Second Vatican Council. Indeed, one of the revisions to the 2018 *ERD* is a much greater reliance on canon law as a source of ethical knowledge.

In the Jesuit tradition, discernment is the art of prayerful decision-making that relies on spiritual practices, including the practices of, we would argue, seeing, judging, and acting from a prayerful perspective informed by scripture, tradition, experience, and reason and science.[45] This approach is clearly reflected in *Octogesima Adveniens* and *Populorum Progressio*.[46] In his commentary on *Amoris Laetitia*, André Vingt-Trois, cardinal archbishop of Paris, writes that *Amoris Laetitia* invites all pastoral workers and, we add, all Christians, to return to "meditating on the message of Christ and the Christian tradition of the family and to seek to understand how this message could help to accompany families in the challenges that face them today."[47] Discernment, Francis writes, requires "humility, discretion, and love for the Church and her teaching, in a sincere search for God's will and a desire to make a more perfect response to it" (*AL*, 300). Discernment is much more than simply following rules and absolute norms and moves us from a deontological-type ethic to a virtue-type ethic, grounded in the theological virtues of faith, hope, charity, compassion, justice, and prudence, that helps us to see and judge from a uniquely Christian perspective to act in a uniquely Christian way. Seeing and judging may lead to acts that follow rules and guidelines presented by the Church or to the act of challenging those rules and guidelines. Authentic discernment and an informed conscience allow for and, as Aquinas insisted in the thirteenth century, sometimes may even demand dissent from Church teaching.[48] Since conscience is a practical judgment that comes at the end of a deliberative process, it necessarily involves the virtue of prudence, by which, according to the *Catechism*, "right reason is applied to action" (1806).

Amoris Laetitia and Virtues

The shift from a focus on rules and acts to a focus on virtue is a third fundamental anthropological and methodological shift in *Amoris Laetitia*. Virtue focuses first on the character of a person rather than on her/his acts, on being rather than doing, but there is still an ongoing dialectic between virtue and acts. Acts are important since they both reflect and, when repeated, shape virtuous character; virtue both manifests and produces itself in acts. In virtue ethics, ethical agents and their characters come first, and their ethical actions come second; *agere sequitur esse*, action follows being.[49] The focus in *Amoris Laetitia* is not on rules and acts but on ways of being in the world, where the person is invited to strive to live a life like Christ in the service of God, spouse, family, neighbor, and society, all the while understanding that God's mercy is infinite if we fall short. Chapter 4 of *Amoris Laetitia*, "Love in Marriage," is a beautiful reflection on Saint Paul's poetic passage on the nature of true love (1 Cor 13:4–7) and the virtues associated with it. Love is patient, directed toward service, generous, forgiving, not jealous, boastful, or rude. It is noteworthy that the virtue of chastity, so central in the traditional Catholic approach to love, sexuality, and marriage, and so often deductively applied as a legalistic submission to the Church's absolute proscriptive laws on sexuality, is mentioned only once in *Amoris Laetitia*, and this in the context of proving "invaluable for the genuine growth of love between persons" (*AL*, 206). Rather than an exclusive focus on chastity, there is a greater focus on the virtues of love (89–164), mercy (27, 47, 300, 306), compassion (28, 92, 308), reconciliation (106, 236, 238), forgiveness (27, 236, 268), and prudence (262).

Prudence is a cardinal virtue that guides all other virtues and is a prerequisite virtue for both conscience and discernment. Aquinas argues, indeed, that it is an essential prerequisite for the possession of all other virtues. It discerns the first principles of morality, applies them to particular situations, and enables conscience to make practical judgments that this is the right thing to do on this occasion and with this good motive (*ST*, I–II, q. 47, a. 6). Prudence is said to be a *cardinal* virtue because it is a *cardo* or hinge around which all other virtues turn, integrating agents and their actions and ensuring that they make the right virtuous choice (*ST*, I, q. 65, a. 1). It is not difficult to see how it is an essential hinge around which the practical judgment of conscience and its right virtuous choice turns.

Pope Francis's Catholic holistic human dignity emphasizes a relational ontology, the authority and inviolability of conscience guided by an evolving understanding of natural law through discernment guided by the virtues, especially the virtue of prudence. This is a very different anthropology than the Catholic sexual human dignity reflected in the *ERD*. It emphasizes a physicalist ontology, focuses on the subservience of conscience to immutable, absolute natural law, and insists that obedience to those norms is the highest virtue.

HUMAN DIGNITY AND THE *ERD*

The tension between Catholic sexual human dignity and Catholic social and holistic human dignity, between a physical and relational ontology, between focus on rules and laws and focus on principles and virtues, and different understandings of conscience is clearly illustrated in the *ERD* and the directive prohibiting the use of artificial contraception within the marital relationship. The introduction to part 4 of the *ERD* states, "The Church cannot approve contraceptive interventions that 'either in anticipation of the marital act, or in its accomplishment, or in the development of its natural consequences, have the purpose, whether as an end or a means, to render procreation impossible.' Such interventions violate 'the inseparable connection, willed by God . . . between the two meanings of the conjugal act: the unitive and procreative meaning'" (*ERD*, 16). Both quotes are taken directly from *Humanae Vitae*, numbers 14 and 12, respectively. This teaching is formulated in directive 52: "Catholic health institutions may not promote or condone contraceptive practices but should provide, for married couples and the medical staff who counsel them, instruction both about the Church's teaching on responsible parenthood and in methods of natural family planning." However, directives 47 and 53 allow exceptions to absolute norms prohibiting direct abortion and direct sterilization, respectively, to treat a serious physical pathology. Though not explicitly stated in the *ERD*, based on these exceptions, one can reasonably conclude that, following *Humanae Vitae* 15, the *ERD* allows the use of "therapeutic means necessary to cure bodily diseases."

There are several points to note regarding Church teaching and the *ERD* and its exception to the absolute norm prohibiting the use of contraceptives to treat a physical pathology. First, although the ontology guiding the *ERD* on contraceptives emphasizes the relational and biological dimensions and the inseparable unitive and procreative meanings of the marital act, there is a clear prioritization of the physical over the relational. On the one hand, no relational considerations can justify the use of contraceptives in the marital relationship. On the other hand, treating a physical pathology can justify the use of contraceptives as long as the intention is to treat the pathology and not to prevent conception. This exception clearly places biological/physical ontology over relational ontology in ethically evaluating the conscience judgment by a married couple on the use of contraceptives.

Second, although Church teaching recognizes the principle of responsible parenthood as a legitimate principle for limiting the number of children a couple chooses to have, this principle translates into the absolute norm prohibiting contraceptives to regulate fertility in the *ERD*. Only "methods of natural family planning" (*ERD*, dir. 52) are allowed to regulate fertility. The *ERD* and its focus on absolute rules and norms reflects Pope John Paul's Catholic sexual human dignity and the obligation of conscience to adhere to these rules and norms. Pope Francis also emphasizes the principle of responsible parenthood. Regarding this principle, he notes that it "requires that husband and wife, keeping a right order of priorities, recognize their own duties towards God, themselves, their families and human society" (*AL*, 222; *HV*, 10), in other words, prioritizing personal and social relational dimensions in the process of discernment, conscience formation, and judgment. Guided by conscience, he states, the couple "will make decisions by common counsel and effort. Let them thoughtfully take into account both their own welfare and that of their children, those already born and those which the future may bring. . . . The parents themselves *and no one else* should ultimately make this judgment in the sight of God" (*AL*, 222; *GS*, 50; emphasis added). Furthermore, "the use of methods based on the 'laws of nature and the incidence of fertility' (*HV*, 11) *are to be promoted*, since 'these methods respect the bodies of the spouses, encourage tenderness between them and favor the education of an authentic freedom'" (*AL*, 222; *CCC*, 2370; emphasis added). *Amoris Laetitia* makes no mention of *Humanae Vitae* 12 or *Familiaris Consortio* 32, both of which specifically condemn artificial contraception in the marital relationship.

Relatio Synodi 58 mentions "natural methods for responsible procreation," but it is noticeably absent from *Amoris Laetitia* itself.[50] Francis references John Paul II's *Familiaris consortio* 14, which lauds children as the "precious gift of marriage" (*AL*, 42), but nowhere does he mention the absolute inseparability of the unitive and procreative meanings of sexual intercourse so emphasized by Paul VI in *Humanae Vitae* 11 and 12 and so central to his banning of all artificial contraception, reiterated in the *ERD*. Without specifically abrogating Paul VI's much-controverted teaching, Francis comes down on what to some is a new but is really an old though recently magisterially ignored Catholic principle of the absoluteness and inviolability of an informed conscience. Decisions about family planning, Francis insists, "fittingly takes place as the result of a consensual dialogue between the spouses." It is a decision that flows from an informed conscience, "which is 'the most secret core and sanctuary of a person' where 'each one is alone with God whose voice echoes in the depth of the heart'" (*AL*, 222; *GS*, 16). The Second Vatican Council taught that the married couple "will make decisions [about the transmission of life] by common counsel and effort. . . . The parents themselves and no one else should ultimately make this judgment in the sight of God" (*AL*, 222; *GS*, 50). Francis reinforces this in his decree that any conscience judgment should ultimately be the decision of the couple based on relational considerations, a decree that does not absolutely forbid contraception and may, in fact, be interpreted to promote it.

The *ERD* and its teaching on contraception is just one example where it has failed to recognize or incorporate Pope Francis's anthropological integration and expansion of Catholic sexual and social human dignity into what we label Catholic holistic human dignity. This is a missed opportunity for the revised *ERD* to move the tradition forward in light of Pope Francis's more comprehensive, comprehensible, and credible definition of human dignity more in line with tradition and the Second Vatican Council than is the absolute pro-scriptions in the *ERD*. Not only does Pope Francis's anthropology demonstrate this integration and expansion, so too does his ethical methodology, which we address in the next chapter.

SUGGESTED READINGS

DeCosse, David E., and Thomas A. Nairn, OFM. *Conscience and Catholic Health Care: From Clinical Contexts to Government Mandates*. Maryknoll, NY: Orbis, 2018.

Francis. *Amoris Laetitia*. Available at https://w2.vatican.va/content/dam/francesco/pdf /apost_exhortations/documents/papa-francesco_esortazione-ap_20160319_amoris -laetitia_en.pdf.

John Paul II. *The Theology of the Body: Human Love in the Divine Plan*. Boston, MA: Pauline Books and Media, 1997.

Rausch, Thomas, SJ, and Roberto Dell'Oro. *Pope Francis on the Joy of Love: Theological and Pastoral Reflections on* Amoris Laetitia. New York: Paulist Press, 2018.

Salzman, Todd A., and Michael G. Lawler. *The Sexual Person: Toward a Renewed Catholic Anthro-pology*. Washington, DC: Georgetown University Press, 2008.

NOTES

1. John Paul II developed this position in a series of talks he gave from 1979 to 1981. These talks are now published as *The Theology of the Body: Human Love in the Divine Plan*, with a foreword by John S. Grabowski (Boston, MA: Pauline Books and Media, 1997), 48, 49.

2. It is important to note that the distinction between biological sex (male/female) and socially constructed gender (masculine/feminine) is frequently absent in Church discus-sions of complementarity. See Susan A. Ross, "The Bridegroom and the Bride: The Theo-logical Anthropology of John Paul II and Its Relation to the Bible and Homosexuality," in *Sexual Diversity and Catholicism: Toward the Development of Moral Theology*, ed. Patricia Beattie Jung with Joseph A. Coray (Collegeville, MN: Liturgical, 2001), 39–59, at 56n5.

3. Ross, "Bridegroom and the Bride"; and David M. McCarthy, "The Relationship of Bodies: A Nuptial Hermeneutics of Same-Sex Unions," in *Theology and Sexuality: Classic and Contemporary Readings*, ed. Eugene F. Rogers (Oxford: Blackwell, 2002), 200–216, at 206–10.

4. John Paul II, "Authentic Concept of Conjugal Love," *Origins* 28 (March 4, 1999): 654–56, at 655. John Paul II, "Letter to Women (27 July 1995)," 7, available at http://www .vatican.va/content/john-paul-ii/en/letters/1995/documents/hf_jp-ii_let_29061995 _women.html.

5. *HV*, 10; see also Pope Pius XII, "The Apostolate of the Midwife," in *The Major Ad-dresses of Pope Pius XII. Vol. I: Selected Addresses*, ed. Vincent A. Yzermans (St. Paul, MN: North Central Publishing, 1961), 169.

6. John Paul II, "Letter to Women," 7. See CDF, "Considerations Regarding Proposals to Give Legal Recognition," 4; *CCC*, 2357.

7. Pope John Paul II, "World Day of Peace" (January 1, 1995), in *The Genius of Women* (Washington, DC: United States Catholic Conference, 1999), 3.

8. Edward Collins Vacek, "Feminism and the Vatican," *Theological Studies* 66, no. 1 (2005): 159–77, at 173–74, referring to John Paul II, "Authentic Concept of Conjugal Love," 655.

9. John Paul II, "Letter to Women," 7.

10. John Paul II, emphasis in original. *FC*, 19. For a response to "ontological complementarity," see Kevin Kelly, *New Directions in Sexual Ethics* (London: Cassell, 1999), 51–52.

11. John Paul II, "Letter to Women," 8; *Mulieris Dignitatem*, 6; John Paul II, "Authentic Concept of Conjugal Love," 655.

12. *FC*, 32; John Paul II, *Evangelium Vitae*, 14. While the falsification of conjugal love specifically addresses contraception in this paragraph, according to magisterial teaching, it applies to reproductive technologies as well. See Congregation for the Doctrine of the Faith, *Donum Vitae: Instruction on Respect for Human Life in Its Origin and on the Dignity of Procreation: Replies to Certain Questions of the Day* (Washington, DC: Office of Publishing and Promotion Services, United States Catholic Conference, 1987).

13. John Paul II, *Theology of the Body*, 387.

14. See Ronald Modras, "Pope John Paul II's Theology of the Body," in *John Paul II and Moral Theology: Readings in Moral Theology No. 10*, ed. Charles Curran and Richard McCormick (New York: Paulist Press, 1998), 149–56. See Lisa Sowle Cahill, "Catholic Sexual Ethics and the Dignity of the Person: A Double Message," *Theological Studies* 50, no. 1 (1989): 120–50, at 145–46; Luke Timothy Johnson, "A Disembodied 'Theology of the Body': John Paul II on Love, Sex, and Pleasure," *Commonweal* 128, no. 2 (January 26, 2001): 11–17; Margaret Farley *Just Love: A Framework for Christian Sexual Ethics* (New York: Continuum, 2006).

15. Karol Wojtyla, *Love and Responsibility* (Boston: Pauline Books and Media, 2013), 229–30.

16. Wojtyla, 53.

17. See also The Pontifical Council for the Family, "Family, Marriage and 'De Facto' Unions," (January 11, 2001): 8, available at http://www.vatican.va/roman_curia/pontif ical_councils/family/documents/rc_pc_family_doc_20001109_de-facto-unions_en.html. According to this statement, biological sex and not cultural gender is the foundation for interpersonal relationships. "According to this ideology [of gender], being a man or a woman is not determined fundamentally by sex but by culture. Therefore, the very bases of the family and inter-personal relationships are attacked."

18. Congregation for Catholic Education, "'Male and Female He Created Them': Towards a Path of Dialogue on the Question of Gender Theory in Education (2 February 2019)," 31, emphasis added, available at https://www.vatican.va/roman_curia/congregations/ccath educ/documents/rc_con_ccatheduc_doc_20190202_maschio-e-femmina_en.pdf.

19. Athalya Brenner, *The Intercourse of Knowledge: On Gendering Desire and 'Sexuality' in the Hebrew Bible* (New York: Brill, 1997), 12.

20. Edward N. Peters, *The 1917 Pio-Benedictine Code of Canon Law* (San Francisco: Ignatius Press, 2001), Can. 1081, 2.

21. See Michael G. Lawler, *Marriage and the Catholic Church: Disputed Questions* (Collegeville, MN: Liturgical Press, 2002), 77–85.

22. See Todd A. Salzman and Michael G. Lawler, *The Sexual Person: Toward a Renewed Catholic Anthropology* (Washington, DC: Georgetown University Press, 2008), 236–58.

23. Charles E. Curran, *Catholic Social Teaching, 1891–Present: A Historical, Theological, and Ethical Analysis* (Washington, DC: Georgetown University Press, 2002), 131.

24. John A. Coleman, "The Future of Catholic Social Thought," in *Modern Catholic Social Teaching: Commentaries and Interpretations*, ed. Kenneth Himes (Washington, DC: Georgetown University Press, 2005), 522–44, at 527–29.

25. International Theological Commission, "In Search of a Universal Ethic: A New Look at Natural Law," May 20, 2009, 55, available at http://www.vatican.va/roman_cu ria/congregations/cfaith/cti_documents/rc_con_cfaith_doc_20090520_legge-naturale _en.html.

26. Brian Stiltner, *Religion and the Common Good* (Lanham, MD: Rowman and Littlefield, 1999), 178.

27. David Hollenbach, "The Catholic University and the Common Good," 1–19, at 2, available at https://www.bc.edu/content/dam/files/offices/mission/pdf1/cu22.pdf.

28. See Mary Elsbernd, "The Reinterpretation of *Gaudium et Spes* in *Veritatis Splendor*," *Horizons* 29, no. 2 (2002): 225–39, at 233–34.

29. Pope Francis, World Day of Peace Message (2017), 5.

30. Pope Francis, Lenten Message (2015).

31. See Donal Dorr, "Solidarity and Integral Human Development," in *The Logic of Solidarity: Commentaries on Pope John Paul II's Encyclical "On Social Concern,"* ed. Gregory Baum and Robert Ellsberg (New York: Orbis, 1989), 143–54.

32. See Basil, *In illud Lucae, PG*, 31, 263; Augustine, *Enarratio in Ps CXLVII*, 12, *PL*, 37, 192; Gregory the Great, *Regulae Pastoralis Liber*, pars. 3, chap. 21, *PL*, 77, 87. There is an ancient Catholic principle, "In extreme necessity all goods are to be shared," but see Aquinas's explanation of how that principle is to be applied in *ST*, II–II, q. 66, a. 7.

33. USCCB, "A Compilation of Quotes and Texts of Pope Francis on Dialogue, Encounter, and Interreligious and Ecumenical Relations," available at http://www .usccb.org/beliefs-and-teachings/ecumenical-and-interreligious/resources/upload /Quotes-of-Pope-Francis-on-dialogue-encounter-ecumenical-and-interreligious-af fairs-12042013.pdf.

34. USCCB.

35. Cindy Wooden, "'*Amoris Laetitia*' at Three Months: Communion Question Still Debated," *National Catholic Reporter*, July 7, 2016, available at https://www.ncronline.org/news /parish/amoris-laetitia-three-months-communion-question-still-debated.

36. Edward Pentin, "Cardinal Parolin: *Amoris Laetitia* Represents New Paradigm, Spirit and Approach," *National Catholic Register* (January 11, 2018), available at http://www .ncregister.com/blog/edward-pentin/cardinal-parolin-amoris-represents-new-paradigm -new-spirit-new-approach.

37. Janssens, "Artificial Insemination," 3–29.

38. For a worldwide sociological survey of Catholic beliefs on a variety of sexual ethical issues, see Univision Communications, *Global Survey of Roman Catholics*, Executive Summary (New York, February 2014), available at http://pelicanweb.org/2014RCSurveyExecutive Summary.pdf.

39. Lizzy Davies, "Pope Francis Tells Atheists to Abide by Their Own Consciences," *The Guardian*, September 11, 2013, available at https://www.theguardian.com/world/2013/sep/11/pope-francis-atheists-abide-consciences.

40. Pope Francis, "Jesus Always Invites Us: He Does Not Impose," *Angelus*, June 30, 2013, available at http://whispersintheloggia.blogspot.com/2013/06/jesus-always-invites-us-he-does-not-impose.html.

41. Elsbernd, "Reinterpretation of *Gaudium et Spes*," 234.

42. See Michael G. Lawler and Todd A. Salzman, "Conscience and Experience: Choosing the True and the Good," *Irish Theological Quarterly* 81, no. 1 (2016): 34–54; David E. DeCosse and Thomas A. Nairn, *Conscience and Catholic Health Care: From Clinical Contexts to Government Mandates* (Maryknoll, NY: Orbis, 2018).

43. Pope Pius X, *Vehementer Nos* (February 11, 1906), 8, available at http://www.vatican.va/content/pius-x/en/encyclicals/documents/hf_p-x_enc_11021906_vehementer-nos.html.

44. See George M. Regan, *New Trends in Moral Theology* (New York: Paulist, 1971), 25.

45. James Martin, "Understanding Discernment Is Key to Understanding *Amoris Laetitia*," *America*, April 8, 2016, available at http://www.americamagazine.org/issue/discernment-key-amoris-laetitia.

46. See Marvin L. Mich, "Commentary on *Mater et Magistra* (Christianity and Social Progress)," in *Modern Catholic Social Teaching*, 191–216, at 198, 203–4. See Allan Figueroa Deck, "Commentary on *Populorum Progressio* (On the Development of Peoples)," in *Modern Catholic Social Teaching*, 292–314, at 299–300.

47. See Anne-Bénédicte Hoffner, "*Amoris Laetitia* Requires an Effort of Formation of Discernment," *LaCroix International* (October 19, 2016), available at https://international.la-croix.com/news/amoris-laetitia-requires-an-effort-of-formation-for-discernment/4085.

48. Thomas Aquinas, *IV Sent.*, dist. 38, q. 2, art. 4.

49. See Daniel Statman, "Introduction to Virtue Ethics," in *Virtue Ethics: A Critical Reader*, ed. Daniel Statman (Washington, DC: Georgetown University Press, 1997), 1–41, at 7; Todd A. Salzman and Michael G. Lawler, *Virtue and Theological Ethics: Toward a Renewed Ethical Method* (Maryknoll, NY: Orbis, 2018).

50. *Relatio synodi*, Vatican City, 2014, 58, available at http://www.vatican.va/roman_curia/synod/documents/rc_synod_doc_20141018_relatio-synodi-familia_en.html.

CHAPTER THREE

Ethical and Methodological Tensions in the *ERD*

In chapter 1, we investigated the sources of ethical knowledge and how different perspectives on the selection, interpretation, prioritization, and integration of the sources lead to tensions in the formulation, interpretation, and application of the *ERD*. In this chapter, we continue the methodological discussion, highlighting tensions in Catholic ethical method and the *ERD* depending on the category of ethical issues—social, sexual, environmental, and health care—and propose a Catholic holistic ethical method that seeks to integrate the best of these methods. We argue that Pope Francis's *Amoris Laetitia, Laudato Si'*, and the Amazon Synod all provide a road map for constructing a Catholic holistic ethical method, a comprehensive, comprehensible, and credible method that can serve as a methodological guide for the revision of the *ERD* and the reformulation or addition of specific directives.

ETHICAL METHOD AND THE *ERD*

We begin our discussion of Catholic ethical method with an interview Pope Francis gave to reporters on his return flight from Africa. When asked if the Church should consider a change in its absolute prohibition of the use of condoms to prevent the spread of HIV/AIDS, the pope responded that the question seemed too small. "I think the morality of the Church on this point finds itself in a dilemma: is it the fifth or the sixth commandment? To defend life, or is the sexual relation open to life? But this is not the problem." The first problem in Africa, and indeed worldwide, is much bigger and more complex than the use of condoms. The first problem is the reality of "denutrition, the exploitation of people, slave labor, lack of drinking water."[1] Condom use may or may not address a part of the human problem, but the greater problem is systemic social injustice and violations of human dignity throughout the world.

The second problem is the relationship between Church law and human dignity. Francis recalled a specious question put to Jesus by a Pharisee: "Tell me master, is it allowed to heal on the Sabbath?" (Matt. 12:10). Jesus answered that any one of them would rescue his sheep on the Sabbath and "of how much more value is a man than a sheep" (12:12). "Do justice" is Francis's answer; "do not think whether it is allowed or not to heal on the Sabbath. And when all these are cured, when there are no injustices in this world, then we can talk about the Sabbath." The pope's response foreshadows a shift in focus in how the hierarchical magisterium and Catholic theological ethicists should prioritize questions relating to social justice, sexual ethics, and health care, and how, therefore, they should approach those questions anthropologically and methodologically. In chapter 2, we responded to the anthropological question and proposed a Catholic holistic human dignity. In this chapter, recognizing an ongoing dialectic between ethical method and the definition of human dignity, we focus on the methodological question.

Pope Francis's reflection on the relationship between HIV/AIDS prevention and the social injustice of poverty highlights some of the ethical methodological inconsistencies, long noted by Catholic ethicists, between Catholic social teaching in documents such as *Populorum Progressio*, Catholic sexual teaching in documents such as Pope Paul VI's *Humanae Vitae*, Catholic health care teaching in documents such as Pope John Paul II's *Evangelium Vitae*, Catholic environmental teaching in Pope Francis's *Laudato Si'*, and the recent Amazon Synod. Three of the four methods are reflected in the *ERD*, which leads to inconsistencies in how Church teaching and the *ERD* formulate and justify specific ethical directives.[2]

Since the Second Vatican Council, Catholic social teaching has been principle focused, relation focused, dynamic, and inductive. Catholic sexual teaching, on the contrary, has continued to be law oriented, act focused, static, and deductive. Ron Hamel lists characteristics of Catholic health care teaching. First, it relies on an act-focused pre–Second Vatican Council method. Second, it weds this act-focused method to a bioethical principles approach, which prioritizes beneficence, nonmaleficence, autonomy, and justice, and is act focused and tends to concentrate on ethical issues at the beginning and end of life. Third, the emphasis is on ethics in the clinical setting. Catholic health care teaching pays little or no attention to social justice and environmental issues, so emphasized by Pope Francis and often driving health care needs. These issues include poverty, housing, environment, violence, and race and gender consider-ations, to name just a few.[3] The *ERD* also fails to address institutional practices that impact the delivery of health care. Among those practices is what Sheri Bartlett Browne calls the "white space" that predominates in Catholic health care institutions in the United States: the lack of racial and cultural diversity that impacts issues such as end-of-life care and hospice.[4] As America becomes a more diverse and less white society, the structures of, and guidelines for, Catholic health care institutions must pay more attention to racial and cultural diversity. Therese Lysaught and Michael McCarthy accurately conclude that Catholic health care has *scotosis*, or a blind spot. It has not "developed the con-ceptual tools [or method] necessary for engaging the social dynamics, largely fraught with injustices, that shape almost every aspect of health care delivery in the US."[5]

We find three ethical methods in the *ERD*, Catholic social, sexual, and health care teaching. Directive 7 of the *ERD* clearly reflects Catholic social teaching: "A Catholic health care institution must treat its employees respectfully and justly. This responsibility includes: equal employment opportunities for anyone qual-ified for the task, irrespective of a person's race, sex, age, national origin, or dis-ability; a workplace that promotes employee participation; a work environment that ensures employee safety and well-being; just compensation and benefits; and recognition of the rights of employees to organize and bargain collectively without prejudice to the common good." Methodologically, this directive is based on Catholic social teaching and promotes the common good. As is often the case, however, there can be a disconnect between recognizing the legitimacy of an ethical principle and applying it in a particular context. Some Catholic health care institutions, for example, resist the formation of unions that ad-vocate for just wages and better working conditions for health care workers.[6]

The *ERD* also includes references to foundational principles in Catholic social teaching: stewardship (*ERD*, 7, 8, 20, 23, dir. 4, 6), subsidiarity (*ERD*, 8), an option for the poor (*ERD*, 8, 23, 27, dir. 3, 42) and the common good (*ERD*, 7, 8, 23, dir. 7, 9). These are important principles that guide the *ERD* in terms of responsibility to provide preferentially for the poor and their health care needs. The *Catechism of the Catholic Church* teaches that "the Church's social teaching proposes principles for reflection; it provides criteria for judgment; it gives guidelines for action" (*CCC*, 2423). This trinity, principles for reflec-tion, criteria for judgment, and guidelines for action, came into Catholic social teaching via Pope Paul VI's *Octogesima Adveniens* in 1971. It was repeated in the CDF's *Instruction on Freedom and Liberation* in 1986 and underscored again a year later in John Paul II's *Sollicitudo Rei Socialis*. This approach to social morality is an authentically established part of the modern Catholic ethical tradition. Pope

John Paul II accentuates this perspective by teaching that, in its social teachings, the Church seeks "to guide people to respond, with the support of rational reflection and of the human sciences, to their vocation as responsible builders of earthly society" (*SRS*, 1). This teaching applies also to any dialogue in a Church that is communion and seeking to responsibly build Catholic health care: Church teaching *guides*; responsible believers *respond*, drawing on Church guidance, their own experience, understanding, and the findings of the human sciences. "Catholic health care should be marked," the *ERD* teaches, "by a spirit of mutual respect among caregivers" (dir. 2) and between caregivers, patients, and the institution.

The principle-oriented, relation-focused, dynamic, and inductive method of Catholic social teaching, which draws from scripture, tradition, science, and experience, is in direct methodological contrast with Catholic sexual teaching, which is law oriented, legalistic, act focused, static, and deductive. The latter teaches absolute norms, positing Church teaching and the local bishop as the sole hermeneutical lens for the selection, interpretation, prioritization, and integration of the sources of ethical knowledge and the absolute requirement of obedience by the individual patient and provider to that teaching as the sine qua non for care and treatment in a Catholic institution, regardless of any informed judgments of conscience to the contrary. The method of Catholic sexual teaching is evident especially in areas of reproductive sexual ethics such as contraception (*ERD*, 16, 30, dir. 48, 52), reproductive technologies (*ERD*, 16, 17, dir. 40, 41), and sterilization (*ERD*, 16, 30 dir. 48, 53, 70). These norms are formulated as absolutes and are applied deductively without any consideration of Catholic social teaching on gender, relational, economic, and cultural variables that confront married couples and may affect, for instance, their ability to practice natural family planning to realize responsible parenthood (dir. 52).

Third, the *ERD* reflects Catholic health care teaching, focusing on individual acts in clinical settings to guide ethical decisions that respect patient autonomy. Directive 56 states, "A person has a moral obligation to use ordinary or proportionate means of preserving his or her life. Proportionate means are those that in the *judgment of the patient* offer a reasonable hope of benefit and do not entail an excessive burden or impose excessive expense on the family or the community" (emphasis added). This directive gives primacy to patient autonomy in discerning and judging whether a means is proportionate and ordinary and, therefore, ethically mandated or disproportionate and extraordinary and, therefore, not ethically mandated. The criterion for determining proportionate or disproportionate means is "reasonable hope of benefit" from means that do not entail "excessive burden," including excessive financial burden to the family or community. This criterion allows for a great deal of fluidity, reflecting the fluidity of Catholic social teaching, on patients' ability to make informed-con-science decisions based on their contextual, relational, cultural, economic, eth-nic, environmental, and spiritual considerations.

Depending on the interpretation and application of specific directives, how-ever, the method of Catholic health care teaching may have limited applicability, even on some end-of-life issues. Following Pope John Paul II's 2004 *Allocution* on artificial nutrition and hydration and the persistent vegetative state patient, directive 58 was revised in the 2009 edition of the *ERD* and remains unchanged in the 2018 edition, to state that ANH is required "in principle . . . for those who cannot take food orally."[7] The obligation extends to PVS patients, "who can reasonably be expected to live indefinitely if given such care" (dir. 58).[8] This "in principle" applies as a general rule and may not be obligatory in certain cir-cumstances, according to the CDF's *Commentary* on the *Allocution*.[9] The USCCB sought clarification from the CDF on exceptions to the general rule, posing the following question: "Is the administration of food and water (whether by natural or artificial means) to a patient in a 'vegetative state' morally obligatory except when they cannot be assimilated by the patient's body or cannot be administered to the patient without causing significant physical discomfort?"[10] The CDF answered in the affirmative.

It is important to note that the two exceptions for not administering ANH to the PVS patient are based on purely physical considerations. The CDF notes that such circumstances will be "rare" and "exceptional" for a patient in a veg-etative state, meaning that, in principle, ANH is morally obligatory for PVS patients.[11] Many Catholic ethicists argue that ANH could be removed from a PVS patient based on the patient's informed, autonomous decision, an advance directive (dir. 25 and 28), and the traditional benefit-burden analysis (dir. 56 and 57).[12] In response to those arguments, Cardinal Rigali and Bishop Lori note that although an advance directive allows for the exercise of "free and informed health care decisions," this applies only to the extent that the decision "does not contradict Catholic principles" (dir. 28).[13] Their interpretation of the *Allocution, Commentary,* and *Responses* require ANH for the PVS patient and would super-sede an autonomous and conscience decision of the patient or the patient's surrogate to be removed from ANH in a PVS since it would contradict the Catholic principle that requires ANH "in principle."

We have two methodological critiques of Rigali and Lori's claim and its implications for dir. 58 that would limit patient autonomy and freedom for the PVS patient or the designated surrogate. The first critique is that what those Catholic principles are in directive 28 is indicated not by an uncritical reading of nontraditional, contingent, conjectural, and therefore non-infallible papal or CDF language, but by a careful hermeneutic of that language in the context of the established universal Catholic moral tradition. Any presumed contradiction, we submit, arises only from a questionable reading of both the traditional and suggested revised Catholic principle guiding the administration of ANH to the PVS patient. The second critique, perhaps more to the methodological point, is that any interpretation of a contradiction of principles arises from the prioritization of a biological ontology over a personal-relational ontology and from the shifting of the freedom to discern the application of Catholic moral principles from a conscientious patient and/or the patient's designated surrogate to a physician, who is mandated to consider only the patient's physical condition and not the patient in his "total and entire life history."[14] A physician who exercises her freedom and medical judgment to declare that ANH "cannot be administered to the patient without causing significant *physical* discomfort" is basing her assessment and judgment on purely physical criteria and, therefore, in relation to the total and entire human person, is acting reductionistically, reflecting the physicalist method of Rigali and Lori.[15] Similarly, from this reductionist perspective, the determination that ANH is morally optional when it "cannot reasonably be expected to prolong life" (dir. 58) reflects a physicalist method since it is based solely on a reductionist clinical judgment of a physician that warrants a decision to remove ANH. In each case, decision-making is removed from the patient or the patient's surrogate based on Rigali and Lori's physicalist method, which emphasizes the judgment of physical discomfort or a prognostic judgment of prolonging life via a reductionist clinical judgment of a physician. This reductionist approach removes significantly or totally patient autonomy to make informed end-of-life decisions. The final phrase of directive 58, however, that can justify the removal of nutrition and hydration is the "ability to prolong life *or* provide comfort" (emphasis added). The inclusion of comfort here clearly enables the patient or surrogate to make the assessment in a holistic manner. The crucial reference to comfort at the end of directive 58 indicates that the reductive focus on physicalism by Rigali and Lori could also be interpreted as a more holistic approach in the *ERD*.

The exclusive prioritization from Rigali and Lori's perspective of physical considerations that trump all other considerations, including relational, psychological, spiritual, moral, and economic ones, indicates the methodological reductionism of their interpretation of the revised benefit/burden principle that emphasizes dying and death primarily as biological and medical events. In Pope John Paul II's *Allocution*, the CDF's *Commentary*, and *Responses*, the moral justification for withholding or withdrawing ANH from the PVS patient is based exclusively on physical criteria, though the *Commentary* does mention that "in principle" does not exclude the physical impossibility of administering ANH, as in the cases of "very remote places" or "extreme poverty." This reductionism is in stark contrast to the original tradition that allowed for a benefit/burden analysis that included physical, emotional, relational, spiritual, and economic considerations and resulted in an autonomous, conscience decision by the patient or the patient's designated surrogate.

From the perspective of Rigali and Lori, then, decision-making and autonomy are removed from the patient, or the patient's advance directive or surrogate, and are placed in the hands of a physician based on the medical diagnosis that a patient is in PVS, no matter whether ANH is excessively burdensome emotionally, relationally, spiritually, or economically. The only *specific* criterion listed that warrants withdrawing ANH for the PVS patient is that its administration causes "significant physical discomfort" (dir. 58). This criterion raises methodological and metaethical concerns about physicalism as an ontological foundation for Rigali and Lori's interpretation of directive 58 rather than personalism.[16]

POPE FRANCIS AND ETHICAL METHOD

There are clear tensions in the *ERD* on the methods of Catholic social, sexual, and health care teachings guiding the formulation, justification, interpretation, and application of specific directives of the *ERD*. We propose Pope Francis's recent work in *Amoris Laetitia*, which proposes "new pastoral methods," in *Laudato Si'*, and in the Amazon Synod, all of which contribute methodological considerations to Catholic health care teaching by investigating the reciprocal relationship between environmental and social ethics and how they impact health care teaching. Francis's methodological contributions and shift in emphases invite a substantial revision of the *ERD* and the formulation of new directives.

Amoris Laetitia and Method

Christoph Cardinal Schönborn, archbishop of Vienna, judges that *Amoris Laetitia* "is the great text of moral theology that we have been waiting for since the days of the [Second Vatican] Council."[17] *Amoris Laetitia* notes that the dialogue during the 2014 and 2015 synods raised the suggestion of "new pastoral methods" tailored to different communities and the marital, familial, and relational realities of those communities (*AL*, 199). It not only affirms but also develops normatively the anthropology of Catholic holistic human dignity and incorporates Catholic social teaching's methodological developments, focusing on inductive reasoning, historical consciousness, and an appreciation of culture, experience, and the sciences. It focuses theologically on scripture and ecclesiology and bridges the traditional disconnect between moral and pastoral theology.[18]

Amoris Laetitia and Philosophical Method

A major methodological shift in *Amoris Laetitia's* sexual teaching is from a deductive to an inductive ethical method. Deductive reasoning begins with an abstract definition of human dignity and universal principles or norms that facilitate or frustrate its attainment. Inductive reasoning, which is a central methodological development in Catholic theological ethics since the Second Vatican Council, begins with particular, cultural, social, relational, and contextual considerations that affect the definition of human dignity, the formulation and justification of norms that facilitate its attainment, and their interpretation and application. Inductive reasoning begins with particular situations in order to attain universal insights.[19] "It is *reductive*," *Amoris Laetitia* (304) notes, "simply to consider whether or not an individual's actions correspond to a general law or rule, because that is not enough to discern and ensure full fidelity to God in the concrete life of a human being." We must begin with the particular contextual reality of the human person to discern what directive applies or what new directive needs to be formulated to address the reality. *Amoris Laetitia* judges that "natural law could not be presented as an already established set of rules that impose themselves a priori on the moral subject" (*AL*, 305). This is the only time that Francis mentions natural law in *Amoris Laetitia* and it is mentioned in the context of a warning against a deductive approach to moral decision-making. It promotes natural law as "a source of objective inspiration for the deeply personal process of making decisions" (*AL*, 305) in all Catholic ethics.

AL cites with approval, for the first time ever in official Catholic sexual teaching, Aquinas's warning that although there is necessity in general principles, the more we descend to matters of detail, the more frequently we encounter defects. "In matters of action, truth or practical rectitude is not the same for all as to matters of detail, but only as to the general principles . . . and the principle will be found to fail as we descend further into detail'" (*AL*, 304; *ST*, I–II, 94, 4). Aquinas's principle has often been cited by Catholic theological ethicists to refute claims to absolute health care and sexual norms. By citing this text from Aquinas, at the very least, *Amoris Laetitia* is cautioning against a deductive, one-rule-fits-all approach to ethical decision-making and is emphasizing an inductive approach and the importance of particular contexts and circumstances.

In its law of gradualness, borrowed from John Paul II and which acknowledges that the human being "knows, loves, and accomplishes moral good by different stages of growth" (*AL*, 295; *FC*, 34), *Amoris Laetitia* recognizes historical consciousness. This is illustrated best in Francis's discussion of the morality of cohabitation. Contrary to the *Final Report* from the synods on the family, which condemns all cohabitation, he makes a distinction between "cohabitation which totally excludes any intention to marry" (*AL*, 53) and cohabitation dictated by "cultural and contingent situations" (*AL*, 294), like poverty, that require a "constructive response" that can lead to marriage when circumstances permit it. We have named the former non-nuptial cohabitation and the latter nuptial cohabitation.[20] Borrowing from Jesus' treatment of the Samaritan woman and applying the law of gradualness, Francis accepts the latter cohabitation "in the knowledge that the human being knows, loves and accomplishes moral good by different stages of growth" (*AL*, 295). The Church must never "desist from proposing the full ideal of marriage, God's plan in all its grandeur," but, aware of all the historical, cultural, psychological, and "even biological" mitigating circumstances, it must also never desist from accompanying "with mercy and patience the eventual stages of personal growth as these progressively appear" (*AL*, 308). The same accompaniment is essential for holistic health care that recognizes structural sin inside and outside Catholic health care institutions and its impact on individuals who require accompaniment.[21] Acknowledging the law of gradualness, an overt expression of historical consciousness, Francis recognizes that some types of cohabitation may be genuinely loving relationships that will grow into marriages. The same law of gradualness may be discerned in conscience to apply to the ethical issue of contraception within marriages.

There is a third shift in philosophical method in *Amoris Laetitia*, dependent on the first and second shifts. Prior to the Second Vatican Council, social, sexual, and medical ethical methods were primarily classicist and deductive: they started with traditional ethical principles, derived absolute norms from those principles, and applied those norms to particular situations, individuals, and acts. *Gaudium et Spes* opened the Church to a historically conscious, inductive approach that starts with the human person in a human situation and works toward specific ethical norms and general ethical principles. It emphasizes that, "thanks to the experience of past ages, the progress of the sciences, and the treasures hidden in the various forms of human culture, the nature of man himself is revealed and new roads to truth are opened" (*GS*, 44). This trilogy of human experience, science, and culture, all sources of ethical knowledge, is paradigmatic for an inductive approach and is widely reflected in *Amoris Laetitia*.

First, *Amoris Laetitia* is based on "the joy of love experienced by families [that] is also the joy of the Church" (*AL*, 1). It is grounded in experience and bases its reflections on both the experience of married life and the sexuality complexly reflected in it, and on socioeconomic factors such as poverty and hunger that so impact it throughout the world (*AL*, 25). Relating human experience to the formulation of norms, Margaret Farley asserts, and we agree, that moral norms cannot become effective in the Church merely "from receiving laws or rules" because reception "entails at the very least a discernment of the meaning of laws and rules in concrete situations." Such discernment requires reflection on human experience—personal, social, and religious—and the social sciences throw revealing light on that experience. We agree wholeheartedly with Farley's further assertion that "it is inconceivable that moral norms can be formulated without consulting the experience of those whose lives are at stake," especially in health care and sexual ethics.[22]

Second, *Amoris Laetitia* recognizes and embraces the importance of particular cultural contexts. This concern for the importance of experiential and cultural particularity was initially evident in the two synods that requested feedback from Catholic faithful on their lived experiences in relationship to Church teaching. Taking this feedback to heart, *Amoris Laetitia* notes that "each country or region . . . can seek solutions [to ethical issues] better suited to its culture and sensitive to its traditions and local needs" (*AL*, 3). The sciences can be helpful for the education, growth, and development of children in families (*AL*, 273, 280). *Gaudium et Spes*'s and *Amoris Laetitia*'s consideration of the importance of experience, science, and culture and the ongoing dialectic between them and scripture and tradition is in contrast to the ecclesial positivism reflected in Catholic sexual and health care teaching. Both of these define *tradition* narrowly as Church teaching and advance the hierarchical magisterium as the sole hermeneutical lens for the selection, interpretation, prioritization, and integration of the sources of ethical knowledge.

AMORIS LAETITIA AND THEOLOGICAL METHOD

AL demonstrates theological development in its use of scripture and offers a unique ecclesiological perspective when approaching marital, sexual ethical issues that have a bearing on Catholic health care teaching. There is a fundamental shift from proscriptive rules to virtues and to scripture as a pedagogical source for virtues in the marital, ethical life. *Amoris Laetitia* also refers to bishops' conferences and how they have responded to particular ethical questions with respect to married and family life (Korean bishops, *AL*, 42; Spanish bishops, *AL*, 32; Mexican bishops, *AL*, 51). Pope Francis has made a concerted effort to empower bishops' conferences, and the consultation of the laity before and during both synods on the family shows his commitment also to the *sensus fidelium* and ecclesial synodality. This consultative process extends beyond "approved authors" specified in the *ERD* to include the faithful and their lived experience in formulating and justifying norms. Such a consultative process expands the current method that limits Catholic health care teaching to the magisterium, which defines *tradition* narrowly as Church teaching, and includes the *sensus fidelium* as an essential dimension of tradition and an important source of ethical knowledge. *Amoris Laetitia*'s process of synodality and discernment promote this expansion of dialogue in the Church.

Discernment is a complex process, which takes time, patience, and a commitment to the kind of charitable dialogue that Pope Francis so appreciated at the 2014 Synod on Marriage and the Family and characterized as "a spirit of collegiality and synodality."[23] Some see a defining characteristic of his papacy as seeking to realize synodality, the ecclesiology of the Second Vatican Council that focuses on journeying together and listening to the input from all quarters of the Church, laity and clerics alike. Synodality requires what both Pope John Paul II and Pope Francis frequently refer to as "dialogue in charity." The two synods, to which *Amoris Laetitia* was a response, modeled this dialogue in a way that synods in the past have not. Synodality and discernment are central and defining dimensions of Pope Francis's papacy and will open the door to further dialogue and development in the Church.

Unfortunately, most bishops in the United States and the USCCB as a body have not embraced synodality as a model of dialogue or acknowledged its fruits. First, even in Pope Francis's synods on the family, the survey sent out by US bishops to collect data from the faithful's perspectives on and experiences of marriage, sexual, and family issues were often screened by bishops. Reports on the surveys by some bishops indicated overwhelming agreement among the faithful on Church teaching on marital and sexual ethical issues, contrary to neutral sociological surveys, which indicate overwhelming disagreement among the faithful on Church teaching on contraception, same-sex marriage, and even abortion.[24] Second, many bishops have not issued statements in their dioceses on *Amoris Laetitia* and its teaching that divorced and remarried Catholics can receive communion following a process of discernment. Where some bishops have issued statements, they promote positions that are selective or even contrary to *Amoris Laetitia* and the *sensus fidelium*.[25] Such episcopal responses to Francis's call for synodality are troubling. They violate the ecclesiology of the Second Vatican Council, ignore the *sensus fidelium*, and disregard the pope's proposal to do things differently in and through synodality and "new pastoral methods."

AMORIS LAETITIA AND NEW PASTORAL METHODS

Pope Francis notes that the two synods preceding *Amoris Laetitia* "raised the need for new pastoral methods . . . that respect both the Church's teaching and local problems and needs" (*AL*, 199). The concept of new pastoral methods draws from both philosophical and theological methods and, for those who interpret *Amoris Laetitia*, highlights a fundamental methodological distinction between moral and pastoral theology, between the objective and subjective realms of morality. Theologian Norbert Rigali addressed this issue thirty years ago, and his observations are especially relevant today in the post–*Amoris Laetitia* era. Rigali argued there has been and, we add, continues to be, a "chasm" for some Catholic ethicists between moral theology and its focus on the objective realm of morality and pastoral theology and its focus on the subjective realm of moral theology. The former emphasizes objective norms, natural law, and magisterial teaching; the latter emphasizes pastoral guidance and subjective conscience. The result is a "two-moral truths theory," one objective and the other subjective.[26] This methodological distinction reflects an ongoing debate on the role and function of conscience in relationship to objective norms and the *ERD*.

It is common in contemporary theological ethics to distinguish between what is called the object orientation and subject orientation of conscience. The former highlights external laws, norms, and directives; the latter highlights conscience's internal discernment, selection, interpretation, and application of norms in light of complex lived reality. On the basis of different methodological perspectives, theological ethicists highlight different orientations when explaining the interrelationship between Church teaching and conscience. Both models of conscience are evident in Catholic tradition. Those who highlight an object orientation, such as Bishop Olmsted, argue that moral norms and directives *must* be followed and, therefore, control the subjective conscience. Those who highlight a subject orientation argue to the contrary that the subjective conscience is free and that, when it makes a moral decision, it *must* take into consideration not only moral norms but also concrete circumstances that can impact their application.

In his *Pastoral Guidelines for Implementing Amoris Laetitia*, Archbishop Charles Chaput of Philadelphia writes that "Catholic teaching makes clear that the subjective conscience of the individual can never be set against objective moral truth as if conscience and truth were two competing principles for moral decision making."[27] In "An Open Letter to Pope Francis," Catholic philosophers Germain Grisez and John Finnis, echoing Chaput's position, list several positions in *Amoris Laetitia* that they judge "contrary to Catholic faith."[28] The *ERD* also prioritizes the object orientation when it states, "Catholic health care does not offend the rights of individual conscience by refusing to provide or permit medical procedures that are judged morally wrong by the teaching authority of the Church" (*ERD*, 8). In one sense, Chaput, Grisez and Finnis, and the *ERD* are correct, there is only one moral truth; conscience and moral truth are not two competing truths but two complementary ways for arriving at that one truth. In another sense, by prioritizing the external, object orientation of a norm or directive, objective moral truth *in itself*, over against the subject orientation of conscience, they are incorrect.[29]

An assertion of an object orientation of conscience, obligating the subjective conscience to obey moral truth without any discernment, is contrary to Catholic teaching. We maintain that forcing that obedience institutionally as a condition for care or treatment in a Catholic health care institution, as does the *ERD*, may be a serious violation of conscience, human dignity, and justice. Any conscience decision must discern moral truth in the subject in light of every relevant circumstance. We are in total agreement with Josef Fuchs and Rigali. Moral truth is not something that objectively exists *in itself apart from* the moral subject but something to be discerned by the moral subject as existing *in myself*. Moral truth is knowledge in the subject of the interrelationship between the moral object and the moral subject; it exists only in the moral subject.[30] Pope Francis seems to defend this kind of prioritization of moral subjects and their consciences. Pope John Paul also seems, at times, to recognize the priority of the subject orientation in relation to the moral object of the act: "In order to be able to grasp the object of an act which specifies that act morally," he writes, "it is therefore necessary to place oneself in the *perspective of the acting person*" (*VS*, 78; emphasis added). This is evident in several different ways in *Amoris Laetitia*.

Speaking of those in the "irregular situation" of being divorced and remarried without annulment, Francis acknowledges that they "can find themselves in a variety of situations, which should not be pigeonholed or fit into overly rigid classifications leaving no room for personal and pastoral discernment" (*AL*, 298). In a footnote that became instantly famous, he cites the Second Vatican Council's judgment that if they take the option of living as brother and sister the Church offers them, "it often happens that faithfulness is endangered and the good of the children suffers" (*AL*, 298, 329).[31] For these reasons, the pope continues, "a pastor cannot feel that it is enough simply to apply [objective] moral laws to those living in 'irregular' situations, as if they were stones to throw at people's lives. This would bespeak the closed heart of one ... judging at times with superiority and superficiality difficult cases and wounded families" (*AL*, 305). Acknowledging the influence on conscience of the various concrete circumstances he has enumerated, the pope advises that subjective "individual conscience needs to be better incorporated into the Church's praxis in certain situations which do not objectively embody our understanding of marriage" (*AL*, 303). His argument, of course, applies not only to marriage, divorce, and remarriage, about which he is specifically speaking, but also to every other concrete ethical situation, including health care ethics.

It is clear that Francis teaches what the Catholic Church teaches but has been reticent to speak about in recent centuries, namely, a subject rather than an object orientation of conscience. To make a genuine conscience judgment, he argues, we need a "harmonious objectivity" in which the internal and external realities of people's concrete lives, which "simply are," are in continuous dialogue with intellectual ideas, which must constantly be "worked out." Intellectual ideas disconnected from concrete realities, Francis judges, "give rise to ineffectual forms of idealism and nominalism, capable at most of classifying and defining, but certainly not calling to [ethical] action. What calls us to [ethical] action are realities illuminated by reason" (*EG*, 232–33).

In the Bishop Olmsted case in Phoenix, it is not that directive 45 has exceptions, which would be the case in an object orientation focus; it is that the directive has nothing to say about the case without subjective understanding and application, which is the case in a subject orientation focus of conscience.[32] In other words, an object orientation begins with some norm and deductively evaluates conscience on whether or not it conforms to the norm and, in the case of the *ERD*, conditions treatment on the basis of that conformity. The burden of proof is on conscience if it claims exceptions to a norm. A subject orientation begins with some concrete situation and discerns inductively what norm applies in the situation and makes a conscience decision in light of that norm and all the morally relevant circumstances. In the case where a norm does not apply, for example, directive 45 prohibiting direct abortion where not performing the abortion would allow the deaths of both a mother of four and her fetus, directive 47 does apply and allows for an operation to cure a "proportionately serious pathological condition of a pregnant woman . . . even if [it] will result in the death of the unborn child." In addition, through the process of consultation and synodality, when complex cases are addressed in light of human experience, the objective norm must be revised to reflect lived experience, just as the objective norm allowing slavery was revised to prohibit slavery or the norm prohibiting usury was revised to allow usury.

Methodologically, Francis's call in *Amoris Laetitia* for "new pastoral methods" that "respect both the Church's teaching and local problems and needs" places him firmly within tradition by prioritizing a subject rather than an object orientation of conscience, overcomes the chasm between moral and pastoral theology, and places a single moral truth where it belongs, in the moral subject's conscience. In other words, "there is not moral law *and* conscience; there is only moral law *of* conscience, the moral law constituting conscience itself."[33] The Church is called to respect this understanding of conscience when it facilitates realizing Catholic holistic human dignity and the common good.

Pope Francis's suggestion of new pastoral methods in *Amoris Laetitia* illuminates a pathway to greater methodological consistency between Catholic social, sexual, and health care ethics by consistently prioritizing the moral subject orientation of a discerning conscience over the moral object orientation of institutional norms external to the subject. Many bishops around the world, including the United States Conference of Catholic Bishops, have resisted this methodological development and, therefore, also the implications of the development for Catholic sexual and health care teaching and for possible revisions of the *ERD*. Francis's development of integral ecology in *Laudato Si'* complements his new pastoral methods recommended in *Amoris Laetitia* and has profound implications for developing an ecological health care ethics.

Laudato Si' and Method

Ron Hamel calls attention to a void in method and content in Catholic health care ethics that does not take ecology into consideration.[34] Following the lead of Howard Brody, he proposes an ecological or environmental health care ethics to complement current Catholic health care ethics.[35] Such a move requires ecological conversion and an integral ecology, both of which are explained in Pope Francis's encyclical on the environment, *Laudato Si'*, and adopted most recently as a method to address environmental, regional, and cultural issues in the Amazon Synod.

LAUDATO SI' AND INTEGRAL ECOLOGY

Jeffrey Sachs, a world-leading economist, has described *Laudato Si'* as "absolutely magnificent." He declares, "I often say that I can assign it to first-year graduate students in earth sciences, biology, theology, diplomacy, or political science. It's so completely holistic that it can be read from all these crucial points of view, so therefore it inspires in its profundity and it speaks to our urgent needs in a very direct way."[36] What makes this encyclical magnificent, we suggest, is its call for an integral ecology and ecological conversion.

Integral ecology is a foundational concept in *Laudato Si'*, which emphasizes that "everything is closely related" (*LS*, 137). To understand Francis's integral ecology, however, we must first understand ecology. The term *ecology* derives from the Greek *oikos* (home), as in the subtitle, *On Care for Our Common Home*, but it has both a narrow biological and a broader theological meaning in *Laudato Si'*. Biologically, it designates the interrelationship between all organisms, including humans, and their natural environment. Theologically, it admires the goodness of God's creation and calls for humans to care for it, guided by the ecological virtues of gratitude for creation, love for creation, solidarity in our common home, mutual responsibility for it, prudent use of it, and justice for all who share it, especially for the poor and vulnerable who are always the most damaged when creation is damaged. It calls also for the recognition of the essential interrelationships that exist between all the organisms that inhabit our common home and for consideration of the social, economic, and political realities that impact these interrelationships.[37] *Laudato Si'* notes that, biologically, "fragmentation of knowledge and the isolation of bits of information can actually become a form of ignorance, unless they are integrated into a broader vision of reality" (*LS*, 139). This is a key insight into the sources of ethical knowledge. A strict hierarchy of those sources, in which *tradition* is narrowly defined as Church teaching and the magisterium serves as the sole hermeneutical lens for the selection, interpretation, prioritization, and integration of the other sources, can lead to a fragmentation of knowledge and can become a form of ecclesial positivism and theological-ethical ignorance promoting *scotosis*. We have seen this historically in Catholic teaching on slavery, usury, and religious freedom and we continue to see it in Church teaching on the role of women in the Church. Integral ecology supports an ongoing dialectic between the four sources of ethical knowledge, especially the contributions of science, to promote the ongoing discernment of ethical truth.

Integral ecology calls for "comprehensive solutions which consider the interactions within natural systems themselves and with social systems" (*LS*, 139). Such comprehensive solutions cannot be found by focusing on social, environmental, and health care crises isolated from one another, for there is "one complex crisis which is both social and environmental." Consequently, "strategies for a solution demand an integrated approach to combating poverty, restoring dignity to the excluded, and at the same time protecting nature" (*LS*, 139). As we have argued, such strategies demand a methodological integration of Catholic social, sexual, health care, and environmental teaching to define human dignity holistically and to formulate, justify, interpret, and apply moral norms to facilitate the attainment of human dignity. Such an integration requires what Pope Francis calls ecological conversion.

Laudato Si' and Ecological Conversion

Pope John Paul II introduced the phrase "ecological conversion" into official Church teaching, intending by it humans' deepened sensitivity to the ecological crisis confronting humanity.[38] In *Laudato Si'* Pope Francis advances "ecological conversion" (*LS*, part 3) as the most fundamental virtue shaping perspectives on the restoration of creation. He notes that many Christians often ridicule concern for the environment or remain passive and do nothing to change their habits to live out their Christian faith consistently. He calls all to "'ecological conversion' whereby the effects of encounter with Jesus Christ become evident in their relationship with the world around them. Living our vocation to be protectors of God's handiwork is essential to a life of virtue; it is not an optional or a secondary aspect of our Christian experience" (*LS*, 217). Francis's *Laudato Si'* focuses on the need for ecological conversion in humans' relationship with and attitude toward the environment. For him, ecological conversion calls for

> a number of attitudes which together foster a spirit of generous care, full of tenderness. First, it entails gratitude and gratuitousness, a recognition that the world is God's loving gift, and that we are called quietly to imitate his generosity in self-sacrifice and good work. . . . It also entails a loving awareness that we are not disconnected from the rest of creatures but joined in a splendid universal communion. As believers, we do not look at the world from without but from within, conscious of the bonds with which the Father has linked us to all beings. By developing our individual, God-given capacities, an ecological conversion can inspire us to greater creativity and enthusiasm in resolving the world's problems and in offering ourselves to God "as a living sacrifice, holy and acceptable" [Rom. 12:1]. (*LS*, 220)

Ecological conversion gives us the courage and insight to ask difficult questions about our current relationship with the environment and to use the sources of ethical knowledge to seek answers to those questions through evaluative judgments that guide human acts. When addressing environmental ethics in general and climate change in particular, ethical method may select all four sources of ethical knowledge and prioritize them in the following order—science, experience, tradition, and scripture—to define human dignity in relation to the environment and to formulate and justify norms and directives that facilitate the attainment of that dignity. This prioritization of the sources, we warn, is not a general ranking of the importance of the sources of ethical knowledge but a ranking of importance for the particular issue of ecological ethics.

Additional methodological considerations in *Laudato Si'* aid in the selection, interpretation, prioritization, and integration of the four sources of ethical knowledge. In the case of climate change and ecological ethics, an inductive approach highlights the importance of science for providing a factual assessment of the environmental situation. This factual assessment is to be prioritized as the point of departure for reflecting on the environmental crisis and its implications for Catholic health care teaching and human dignity and for formulating a normative response. Contextual theology highlights the cultural, historical, and socioeconomic challenges that confront attempts to respond to the climate crisis. The virtues of love and care will have very different normative implications for environmental ethics in a country like the United States, which has the economic and technological resources to effect climate change nationally and internationally, compared to a country like Sudan, which has limited economic and technological resources to effect climate change. The ability to respond to particular ethical issues, especially as these relate to health care, is always very much context dependent. The four sources of ethical knowledge combine to provide an evaluative perspective in which to judge the current ecological crisis in order to act responsibly toward it and to justly address it. Moral conversion, the shift from self-satisfaction to value satisfaction, reveals different values and different ecological virtues to help realize those values.

Among the "sound virtues" that complement ecological conversion, we name prudence, responsibility, courage, humility, honesty, care, faith, hope, love, solidarity, subsidiarity, and reconciliation, all of which pervade *Laudato Si'*. Although we have focused on ecological conversion as the virtuous perspective to address the ecological crisis and to complement the methods of Catholic social, sexual, and health care teachings, Pope Francis has recourse to other virtues that complement conversion and highlight the radical response individuals and local, national, and international communities must take to address the crisis. He voices a particularly urgent moral imperative, grounded in the imitation of Jesus, to respond to this issue in faith and humility.

> Various convictions of our faith . . . can help us to enrich the meaning of this conversion. These include the awareness that each creature reflects something of God and has a message to convey to us, and the security that Christ has taken unto himself this material world and now, risen, is intimately present to each being, surrounding it with his affection and penetrating it with his light. Then too, there is the recognition that God created the world, writing into it an order and a dynamism that human beings have no right to ignore. We read in the Gospel that Jesus says of the birds of the air that "not one of them is forgotten before God" (Lk 12:6). How then can we possibly mistreat them or cause them harm? I ask all Christians to recognize and to live fully this dimension of their conversion. (*LS*, 221)

Focusing on the virtue of care, *Laudato Si'* addresses the need to protect and preserve vital values, especially the human dignity of the poor who suffer the most from any environmental damage. The two assaults on vital human values, climate change and environmental pollution, cause numerous health hazards and millions of premature deaths across the world (*LS*, 20). They also cause the ongoing extinction of plants and animals, which unbalances the ecosystem on which all life depends (*LS*, 36). *Laudato Si'* highlights also another vital value, the interrelationship and interdependence of all creation. "Because all creatures are connected, each must be cherished with love and respect, for all of us as living creatures are dependent on one another" (*LS*, 42). When this relationship is threatened, as it is currently threatened, humans can attempt to compensate for the imbalance through science and technology, but these interventions have unforeseen consequences on the ecological system. A just response to protect vital values must be twofold. Humans must immediately cease assault on the environment with pollution and toxic waste and allow it to heal, and they must do so with technological and scientific solutions that do not further destabilize an already unstable ecosystem. This requires careful planning and national and international cooperation to address very complex issues.

Pope Francis's focus on virtue, in *Amoris Laetitia* with respect to marriage and family and in *Laudato Si'* with respect to the ecological crisis, is a profound methodological development in Catholic Church teaching. Catholic social and ecological teachings have often been ethically evaluated in official Church state-ments from a virtuous perspective, but Catholic sexual teaching and much of health care teaching have focused on individuals, acts, and absolute norms that proscribe particular acts and have neglected a consideration of the environment in Church teaching. Most recently, the Amazon Synod, accurately described as "a son, a daughter, of *Laudato si'*," has sought to "practice what [*Laudato Si'*] preached regarding 'integral ecology' . . . care for our common home."[39] It em-phasizes and expands the call to conversion.[40]

Pope Francis, the Amazon Synod, and Ethical Method

The Amazon Synod incarnates and expands the messages of *Laudato Si'* on integral ecology and ecological conversion. Michael Cardinal Czerny of the Vatican Office for Promoting Integral Development judges that conversion is at the very heart of the Amazon Synod, suggesting "New Paths for the Church and Integral Ecology." The new paths are conversion made concretely manifest. Without conversion, there are no new paths; the Church merely repeats what it has done before without any real change. With the Amazon burning, things have to change, there has to be both social and personal change. There have to be new paths and new responses to new problems. The synod highlights four types of conversion.

First, echoing the urgent call of *Laudato Si'*, the synod calls for ecological con-version. Cardinal Czerny points out that individually, communally, nationally, and internationally too many have not fully grasped the gravity of the ecolog-ical crisis. Among those who have not fully grasped the gravity of the crisis are the bishops of the USCCB. *Laudato Si'* was published in May 2015, and to date there has not been any significant discussion of it among many individual bishops and at the USCCB. At their most recent meeting in November 2019, Cardinal Daniel DiNardo of Galveston-Houston blithely declared that global warming was an important but not an urgent issue, and the body of bishops declared tiredly again that abortion was their "preeminent priority."[41] This flies in the face of Pope Francis's clear teaching in his apostolic exhortation *Gaudete et Exsultate*.

> Our defense of the innocent unborn needs to be clear, firm, and passionate, for at stake is the dignity of a human life, which is always sacred and demands love for each person, regardless of his or her stage of development. Equally sacred, however, are the lives of the poor, those already born, the destitute, the abandoned and the underprivileged, the vulnerable infirm and elderly exposed to covert euthanasia, the victims of human trafficking, new forms of slavery, and every form of rejection. (*GE*, 101)

Francis's teaching is an echo of the "consistent ethic of life" teaching of the late Joseph Cardinal Bernardin of Chicago, which calls for the equal protection of the life and dignity of every human being, born and as yet unborn. Sadly, neither Cardinal Bernardin nor Pope Francis have made much impression on the bishops of the United States, and ecological conversion in America must begin with its bishops. Since the USCCB is unwilling to prioritize ecological conversion, it is not surprising that an ethical concern for the environment and its impact on health care is nowhere recognized in the *ERD*. In 2018 we judge this unconscionable and in serious need of correction.

Second, but important, is pastoral conversion, which is reflected in Pope Francis's "new pastoral methods" in *Amoris Laetitia*. The Church tries to do better, but as conditions in the world change—and they have changed radically in light of climate change—the Church must change as well and cannot continue doing things the same way it has in the past. Pastoral conversion highlights dialogue or synodality among all the faithful, inductive reasoning, and historical consciousness, grounded in human experience and science, to inform and transform tradition in a new world context that responds to lived reality, especially that of the poor.

Third, cultural conversion requires that cultural differences need to be embraced and respected. Cultural conversion requires inculturation, the incarnation of the Gospel in the indigenous cultures. The Church must avoid "colonial-style evangelization" and "proselytism" and instead prioritize "an inculturated proclamation that promotes a Church with an Amazonian face, with full respect for and parity with the history, the culture, and the lifestyle of the local populations."[42] As its population becomes more diverse, this emphasis on respect for cultural diversity and the cultural conversion it requires must be incorporated in the United States as much as in Amazonia. The Church must move believers away from an exclusive focus on ideological disagreements and culture wars and move them toward becoming interculturally respectful. By focusing "preeminently" on culturally divisive issues like abortion, same-sex marriage, and religious freedom, the leadership of the Catholic Church in the United States has helped foster ideological and cultural divisions that actually stifle and prevent cultural conversion.

The fourth conversion is synodality conversion. Synodality is the process of journeying together in discernment and conversion to learn better as a communion Church. It necessarily requires participation of all Catholics in the synodal process, especially those who are allowed little or no voice: the poor, women, "unapproved authors," and a host of others. Synodality is based on listening, reflecting, and praying together as a communion Church to discern responses to the complex problems facing human beings and the Church. The USCCB's earlier documents *Economic Justice for All* and *The Challenge of Peace* were produced via a synodal way of being Church, but in recent years the USCCB has moved away from synodality. The recent USCCB document on racism consulted with victims of racism, but it did not consult with two of the leading theologians writing on theology and race because their positions on women in the Church and on sexual issues were controversial.[43] In the *ERD* it violates synodality by consulting only with "approved authors" who defend Church teaching. Such a narrow focus on hearing only voices that affirm Church teaching respects neither the vocation of Catholic theologians nor the visions of *Gaudium et Spes* and *Amoris Laetitia*.[44]

CATHOLIC HOLISTIC ETHICAL METHOD: A PROPOSAL

In conclusion, we propose a Catholic holistic ethical method (CHEM) that includes the following dimensions. First, it must be grounded in what we called in chapter 1 Catholic holistic human dignity, introduced by Pope Francis in *Amoris Laetitia* and defined as an integration and expansion of Catholic social and sexual human dignity. This holistic human dignity, we believe, lays the foundation for all Catholic ethical teaching. Our definition of it is historically conscious and developmental, just as all knowledge is historically conscious and developmental. Second, Catholic holistic human dignity and CHEM must be in ongoing dialogue since knowledge and understanding of one shape knowledge and understanding of the other. Third, CHEM must incorporate synodality as its preferred process of discernment. Fourth, CHEM must be committed to the common good and its various principles, especially a preferential option for and accompaniment of the poor and the environment. Fifth, CHEM must be inductive and contextual. Sixth, in CHEM the shift in focus from rules to virtues is crucial and requires substantial revision of norms, principles, and directives in the *ERD* in light of that shift.

Seventh, CHEM must recognize personal and structural sin and how these are manifested individually and institutionally. In its recent letter on racism, the USCCB uses the language of structural sin, but it fails to grasp how structures impact individual decisions. This failure is evident in many of the absolute norms of Catholic health care ethics. Focusing on structures of sin and their impacts, environmental deregulation that negatively affects the environment and directly affects community health, must be recognized and challenged. In the *ERD* and its other statements, the USCCB must name and engage the reality of structural sin and draw out its ethical implications and how it frustrates human dignity. Eighth, ongoing openness to pastoral, ecological, synodal, and cultural conversion are essential for discernment and accompaniment. Ninth, reinstating the authority, primacy, and inviolability of an informed conscience, and integrating the object and subject orientations of conscience, is essential to Catholic holistic human dignity anthropologically and to Catholic holistic ethical method methodologically. Tenth, CHEM must avoid a siloed approach to ethics and be cognizant of the interrelatedness of social, sexual, environmental, health care, and all other ethics. Eleventh, it must embrace a dialectical approach to the four sources of ethical knowledge and abandon a narrow, hierarchical approach to them in which tradition is narrowly defined as Church teaching and the hierarchical magisterium serves as the exclusive authority for the selection, interpretation, prioritization, and integration of the four sources. Working out a CHEM and its anthropological and normative implications will be an ongoing process and will require conscientious attention from all levels of the Church in ongoing dialogue with all people of good will and their cultural and contextual realities. We illustrate the normative implications of CHEM with two examples.

Toward a Catholic Environmental Health Care Ethic

Integrating various ethical methods into Catholic health care teaching calls for substantial additions to that teaching in general and to the *ERD* in specific. Hamel suggests specific ways such an integration informs an environmentally sound health care ethics. First and most basically, Catholic health care teaching should emphasize energy conservation by using renewable energy sources and efficient technology in Catholic health care institutions. This will help to reduce carbon emissions and, with concerted efforts institutionally, nationally, and internationally, slow down the effects of climate change. Second, it should promote waste management through reusing or recycling products. Third, creating more efficient and environmentally responsible food production, processing, packaging and distribution can cut down on waste. Pope Francis argues that "to throw food away is to throw people away. . . . It is scandalous today not to notice how precious food is as a good, and how so much good ends up so badly."[45] There is immense food waste in health care facilities. Fourth, health care institutions use more chemicals than any other industry, many of them damaging to both humans, especially vulnerable humans, and the environment. Catholic health care institutions can reduce their use of harmful chemicals by switching to environmentally friendly cleaning products, reducing the use of products with DHEP and PVC, using furniture and carpeting with no harmful chemicals, and eliminating the use of products containing mercury.

Fifth, in the building or renovation of Catholic health care facilities, design, materials, and construction should emphasize sustainability. This includes recycling safe and reusable materials, optimizing energy performance, and reducing harmful chemicals. Design should be attentive to holistic patient care and may include natural light, green areas such as gardens and play areas, and water-efficient landscaping. Sixth, Catholic health care institutions should advocate for legislation that promotes sustainability and energy-efficient city planning and construction. This planning should focus especially on poor areas that have fewer green spaces, experience higher violence and trauma, often serve as dumping grounds for dangerous chemical waste, and lack adequate access to healthy foods. Social advocacy, especially on behalf of the poor, recognizes *Laudato Si's* call for an integrated social and environmental ethic that extends to Catholic health care teaching.[46] The *ERD* should reflect Pope Francis's environmental teaching and ethical methods that draw a clear correlation between environment and health and provide a fruitful landscape for developing a Catholic environmental health care ethic.

THE INTEGRATION OF ETHICAL METHODS AND THEIR IMPACT ON THE *ERD*

Our second example calls for substantial revisions to Catholic sexual and health care teachings and for specific directives in the *ERD* in light of Pope Francis's new pastoral methods. It calls also for greater methodological integration of Catholic social, sexual, environmental, and health care teachings. An essential methodological consideration in *Amoris Laetitia*, *Laudato Si'*, and the Amazon

Synod that brings together Catholic social, environmental, and sexual teaching and has implications for Catholic health care teaching is the recognition of poverty and its profound impact on ethical decisions. Socioeconomic and environmental realities profoundly affect human relationships, and these impacts are often overlooked in Church teaching that proposes norms that are one-size-fits-all. This impact was illustrated in an incident on Pope Francis's visit to the Philippines in January 2015.

On his visit, a former homeless girl, Glyzelle Palomar, gave a heart-wrenching address to the pope and some thirty thousand young people gathered for Filipino youth Sunday. In that address, she burst into tears recounting her experience of homelessness: "There are many children neglected by their own parents. There are also many who became victims and many terrible things happened to them like drugs or prostitution. Why is God allowing such things to happen, even if it is not the fault of the children? And why are there only very few people helping us?"[47] Pope Francis responded to her with his characteristic compassion, imploring Christians to learn how to weep in solidarity with the most vulnerable in society.

What was left unaddressed in both the pope's and the Philippine bishops' responses to Glyzelle's plight, and that of countless others like her around the world, is the correlation between poverty and homelessness, especially among children, and the rigid stance of many bishops, including those of the Philippines, who stridently resist the legalization of birth control in the country. A Guttmacher Institute study indicates that 50 percent of all pregnancies in the Philippines are unintended, and 90 percent of these unintended pregnancies are due to a lack of access to birth control.[48] Only in 2012 did Filipino lawmakers pass a bill for free family planning and access to contraceptives, legislation that the bishops fiercely resisted and continue to resist.[49] On the flight home from the Philippines, Francis reiterated the Church's stance against artificial birth control and defended natural family planning. He also recounted an encounter he had with a pregnant Filipino woman who had seven children. He called this irresponsible and commented, "Some think . . . that in order to be good Catholics we have to be like rabbits—but no."[50] Though we commend the pope for advocating responsible parenthood, we respectfully disagree with Church teaching that natural family planning is the *only* ethically legitimate method for realizing responsible parenthood.

There seems to be a surprising unawareness on the part of the pope and bishops around the world of how patriarchal culture, gender norms, familial relations and socioeconomic and political factors impact reproductive decisions in marriages. This unawareness is a reflection of the fundamental methodological distinction between Catholic social and sexual ethics, the former prioritizing the subject orientation of conscience and offering moral principles for the personal judgment of an informed conscience following careful discernment, the latter prioritizing the object orientation of conscience and offering absolute moral norms for obedience, like the *ERD*'s directive that Catholic institutions "may not promote or condone contraceptive practices" (*ERD*, dir. 52). An integrated methodological approach that prioritizes moral subject orientation would offer a general principle, responsible parenthood, and allow a married couple to work out how to realize this responsible parenthood through discerning and informed consciences that consider all the gender, social, economic, and environmental circumstances. Pope Francis seems to be moving in this direction in *Amoris Laetitia* when he emphasizes that a married couple should make reproductive decisions with an informed conscience based on the principle of responsible parenthood and their particular circumstances, including "the material and the spiritual conditions of the times as well as of their state in life." He concludes that "the parents themselves and no one else should ultimately make this judgment in the sight of God" (*AL*, 222; *GS*, 50). To realize responsible parenthood, "the use of methods based on 'the laws of nature and the incidence of fertility' are to be promoted" (*AL*, 222). A couple should decide on reproductive decisions in conscience, and nowhere in *Amoris Laetitia* is *Humanae Vitae*'s absolute condemnation of artificial contraception cited. Natural methods of fertility regulation are promoted but not absolutely required.

This represents a fundamental shift in Church teaching on decisions about artificial contraception. Such decisions should be guided by the principle of responsible parenthood in light of material and spiritual considerations. Pope Francis seems to have expanded Church teaching on the method for the selection, interpretation, prioritization, and integration of the four sources of ethical knowledge with regard to the sexual ethical issue of fertility regulation. His expansion includes the authority and inviolability of an informed conscience, which reflects a broader understanding of tradition to include the *sensus fidelium* and the lived experience of couples and the material, economic, and environmental conditions that affect their ability to raise children. This is a fundamental methodological shift in how Church teaching has approached the sources of ethical knowledge with respect to Catholic sexual teaching, integrating it with Catholic social teaching and pointing it toward new pastoral methods. This shift has profound implications also for Catholic health care teaching and the *ERD*. We agree fully with Pope Francis on the requirement of first meeting basic needs, social issues relating to the fifth commandment, before we talk about "the Sabbath," in this case health care and sexual issues relating to the sixth commandment. *Amoris Laetitia* makes some progress in integrating Catholic social and sexual teaching, such as its treatment of fertility regulation and economic-driven cohabitation where "material poverty drives people into *de facto* unions" (*AL*, 294) but, we suggest, more integration is needed.

This integration has profound implications for how we consider ethical truth, how we formulate and justify norms to guide conscience, and how we navigate disagreements between Church teaching and informed consciences in Catholic health care institutions. First, it is the role and inviolable authority of conscience to determine whether or not a norm has anything to say about a particular life situation. Highlighting irregular relational situations, Pope Francis seems to indicate that not only is the situation irregular but the norm guiding the situation is as well, and personal conscience must discern which norm to select and how to interpret and apply it in any given situation. In the case of the divorced and remarried without an annulment, for example, it is not the case that a couple may be permitted to take communion as an exception to the general norm but that the general norm itself does not apply in all the specific situations of divorced and remarried couples. Second, as irregular situations gradually become regular, as is now the case with cohabiting couples already committed to marry one another, so-called nuptial cohabitors, and couples practicing artificial contraception in their marital relationship, there may need to be an "organic development of doctrine" that fundamentally transforms the doctrine, similar to the transformation of the doctrines on slavery, usury, and religious freedom.[51] Even though at this point *Amoris Laetitia* changes no specific Catholic doctrines, its anthropological and methodological developments lay a firm foundation for an organic transformation of doctrine, in much the same way as Pope John XXIII's encyclical *Pacem in Terris* laid a firm foundation for the Second Vatican Council's transformation of the doctrine of religious freedom in *Dignitatis Humanae*.[52]

SUGGESTED READINGS

Curran, Charles E. *Catholic Social Teaching: A Historical, Theological, and Ethical Analysis.* Washington, DC: Georgetown University Press, 2002.

Fuchs, Joseph. *Christian Morality: The Word Becomes Flesh.* Dublin: Gill, 1987.

Lysaught, M. Therese, and Michael McCarthy, eds. *Catholic Bioethics and Social Justice: The Praxis of US Health Care in a Globalized World.* Collegeville, MN: Liturgical Press, 2018.

O'Connell, Gerard. "'*Amoris Laetitia*' Represents an Organic Development of Doctrine, 'Not a Rupture.'" *America* (April 8, 2016).

Rigali, Norbert. "The Unity of Moral and Pastoral Truth." *Chicago Studies* 25 (1986): 224–32.

Salzman, Todd A., and Michael G. Lawler. "*Amoris Laetitia*: Towards a Methodological and Anthropological Integration of Catholic Social and Sexual Ethics." *Theological Studies* 79, no. 3 (2018): 634–52.

NOTES

1. Gerard O'Connell, "Pope Francis on Paris Climate Change Summit: 'It's Either Now or Never,'" *America*, November 30, 2015, available at https://www.americamagazine.org/content/dispatches/popes-press-conference-flight-bangui-rome.

2. See Curran, *Catholic Social Teaching*. See Salzman and Lawler, "*Amoris Laetitia*," 634–52.

3. On poverty, housing, and environment, see Ron Hamel, "A Call to Conversion: Toward a Catholic Environmental Bioethics and Environmentally Responsible Health Care," in *Catholic Bioethics and Social Justice: The Praxis of US Health Care in a Globalized World*, ed. M. Therese Lysaught and Michael McCarthy (Collegeville, MN: Liturgical Press, 2018), 235–52. On violence, see Michelle Byrne, Virginia McCarthy, Abigail Silva, and Sharon Homan, "Health Care Providers on the Frontline: Responding to the Gun Violence Epidemic," in Lysaught and McCarthy, *Catholic Bioethics and Social Justice*, 31–45. On race and gender considerations, see David R. Williams, Manuela V. Costa, Adebola O. Odunlami, Selina A. Hohammed, "Moving Upstream: How Interventions That Address the Social Determinants of Health Can Improve Health and Reduce Disparities," *Journal of Public Health Management and Practice* 14, no. 6 (November 2008): S8-S17.

4. See Sheri Bartlett Browne, "Racial Disparities at the End of Life and the Catholic Social Tradition," in Lysaught and McCarthy, *Catholic Bioethics and Social Justice*, 143–60.

5. Lysaught and McCarthy, *Catholic Bioethics and Social Justice*, 2–3. See also Lisa Sowle Cahill, *Theological Bioethics: Participation, Justice, and Change* (Washington, DC: Georgetown University Press, 2005).

6. See Daniel Dwyer, "Unions in Catholic Health Care: A Paradox," in Lysaught and McCarthy, *Catholic Bioethics and Social Justice*, 165–77.

7. Pope John Paul II, "To the Participants in the International Congress on 'Life-Sustaining Treatments and Vegetative State: Scientific Advances and Ethical Dilemmas,'" (2004), available at www.vatican.va/holy_father/john_paul_ii/speeches/2004/march/documents/hf_jp-ii_spe_20040320_congress-fiamc_en.html.

8. Although the ERD uses the language of Persistent Vegetative State, the scientific and medical literature often distinguish between "persistent," a *diagnosis* that "refers only to a condition of past and continuing disability with an uncertain future," and "permanent," a *prognosis* that "implies irreversibility." A person moves from a persistent to a permanent vegetative state "when the diagnosis of irreversibility can be established with a high degree of clinical certainty" (Multi-Society Task Force on PVS, "Medical Aspects of the Persistent Vegetative State," *NEJM* 330 [1994]: 1499–1508, at 1501). We believe that the ERD would be more accurate to refer to a permanent rather than a persistent vegetative state.

9. CDF, *Commentary*, September 16, 2007, available at http://www.vatican.va/roman_curia/congregations/cfaith/documents/rc_con_cfaith_doc_20070801_nota-commento_en.html.

10. CDF, "Responses to Certain Questions of the United States Conference of Catholic Bishops concerning Artificial Nutrition and Hydration," September 16, 2007 (emphasis in original), available at www.vatican.va/roman_curia/congregations/cfaith/documents/rc_con_cfaith_doc_20070801_risposte-usa_en.html.

11. CDF, *Commentary*.

12. John J. Hardt and Kevin O'Rourke, OP, "Nutrition and Hydration: The CDF Response, in Perspective," *Health Progress* (November–December 2007), available at https://www.chausa.org/publications/health-progress/article/november-december-2007/nutrition-and-hydration; and Kelly et al., *Contemporary Catholic Health Care Ethics*, 193–204.

13. Cardinal Justin F. Rigali and Bishop William E. Lori, "On Basic Care for Patients in the 'Vegetative' State," *Health Progress* 89, no. 3 (May–June 2008), available at https://www.chausa.org/publications/health-progress/article/may-june-2008/on-basic-care-for-patients-in-the-%27vegetative%27-state.

14. See Todd A. Salzman and Michael G. Lawler, "Karl Rahner's Theology of Dying and Death: Normative Implications for the Permanent Vegetative State Patient," *Irish Theological Quarterly* 77, no. 2 (May 2012): 141–64. Karl Rahner, SJ, "The Liberty of the Sick, Theologically Considered," in *Theological Investigations*, vol. 17, trans. Margaret Kohl (New York: Crossroad, 1981), 100–113, at 107.

15. CDF, "Responses."

16. We are indebted to Gerard Magill for his helpful suggestions in this section.

17. Cindy Wooden, "'*Amoris Laetitia*' at Three Months: Communion Question Still Debated," *National Catholic Reporter*, July 7, 2016, available at https://www.ncronline.org/news/parish/amoris-laetitia-three-months-communion-question-still-debated.

18. Norbert Rigali, SJ, "The Unity of Moral and Pastoral Truth," *Chicago Studies* 25 (1986): 224–32, at 225.

19. See Richard B. Miller, *Casuistry and Modern Ethics: A Poetics of Practical Reasoning* (Chicago: University of Chicago Press, 1996).

20. Michael G. Lawler and Gail S. Risch, "A Betrothal Proposal," *U.S. Catholic* 72 (June 2007): 18–22, available at http://www.uscatholic.org/life/2008/06/a-betrothal-proposal.

21. See Lysaught and McCarthy, *Catholic Bioethics and Social Justice*, part 1, "Accompanying Vulnerable Communities."

22. Margaret A. Farley, "Moral Discourse in the Public Arena," in *Vatican Authority and American Catholic Dissent*, ed. William W. May (New York: Crossroad, 1987), 168–86, at 177.

23. See Pope Francis, "Address of His Holiness Pope Francis for the Conclusion of the Third Extraordinary General Assembly of the Synod of Bishops, (October 18, 2014)," available at https://w2.vatican.va/content/francesco/en/speeches/2014/october/documents/papa-francesco_20141018_conclusione-sinodo-dei-vescovi.html.

24. See Christine Schenk, "Underreported Survey Responses for Synod on the Family a Valuable Tool for Vatican," *National Catholic Reporter*, June 19, 2014, available at https://www.ncronline.org/blogs/simply-spirit/underreported-survey-responses-synod-family-valuable-tool-vatican.

25. See Crux Staff, "Chaput Says for Communion, Divorced/Remarried Must Live Chastely," *Crux*, July 5, 2016, available at https://cruxnow.com/church-in-the-usa/2016/07/chaput-says-divorcedremarried-must-renounce-sex-get-communion/.

26. Rigali, "Unity of Moral and Pastoral Truth," 224–25.

27. Archdiocese of Philadelphia, "Pastoral Guidelines for Implementing

Amoris Laetitia," July 1, 2016, available at http://archphila.org/wp-content/uploads/2016/06/AOP_AC-guidelines.pdf.

28. John Finnis and Germain Grisez, "An Open Letter to Pope Francis," *First Things*, December 9, 2016, available at https://www.first things.com/web-exclusive/2016/12/an -open-letter-to-pope-francis. For a response to Finnis and Grisez, see Todd A. Salzman and Michael G. Lawler, "Critics of Pope Francis and *Amoris Laetitia*," *New Theology Review* 30, no. 2 (2018): 43–54.

29. Josef Fuchs, *Christian Morality: The Word Becomes Flesh* (Dublin: Gill, 1987), 125.

30. Rigali, "Unity of Moral and Pastoral Truth," 225–27.

31. See *GS*, 51.

32. Rigali, "Unity of Moral and Pastoral Truth," 229.

33. Rigali, 226.

34. Hamel, "Call to Conversion."

35. Howard Brody, *The Future of Bioethics* (New York: Oxford University Press, 2009).

36. Cited in Christopher White, "Economist Sachs Acts as Pope's Cheerleader on '*Laudato Si*,'" *Crux*, June 30, 2018, available at https://cruxnow.com/vatican/2018/0 6/economist-sachs-acts-as-popes-cheerleader-on-laudato-si/.

37. Celia Deane-Drummond, "*Laudato Si*' and the Natural Sciences: An Assessment of the Possibilities and Limits," *Theological Studies* 77, no. 2 (2016): 392–93.

38. Pope John Paul II, "General Audience (Wednesday 17 January 2001)," available at http://w2.vatican.va/content/john-paul-ii/en/audiences/2001/documents/hf_jp-ii _aud_20010117.html.

39. Luke Hansen, "In the Amazon, Pope Francis Is Setting the Agenda for a New Kind of Synod," *America*, September 12, 2019, available at https://www.americamagazine.org /faith/2019/09/12/amazon-pope-francis-setting-agenda-new-kind-synod.

40. "Amazon Synod: The Church Committed to Be an Ally with Amazonia," *Vatican News*, October 26, 2019, available at https://www.vaticannews.va/en/vatican-city/news /2019-10/amazon-synod-final-document.html.

41. See Thomas Reese, "Abortion Preeminent Issue, Global Warming Not Urgent, Say Bishops," *National Catholic Reporter*, November 14, 2019, available at https://www.ncron line.org/news/accountability/signs-times/abortion-preeminent-issue-global-warming -not-urgent-say-bishops.

42. "Amazon Synod," *Vatican News*.

43. USCCB, "Open Wide Our Hearts: The Enduring Call to Love: A Pastoral Let-ter against Racism" (Washington, DC: USCCB, 2018), available at http://www.usccb.org /issues-and-action/human-life-and-dignity/racism/upload/open-wide-our-hearts.pdf.

44. See Salzman and Lawler, "Theologians and Magisterium," 7–31.

45. Devin Watkins, "Pope Francis: 'Food Banks Fight Both Hunger and Waste," *Vati-can News*, May 18, 2019, available at https://www.vaticannews.va/en/pope/news/2019-05 /pope-francis-european-food-banks-federation-hunger-waste.html.

46. See Hamel, "Call to Conversion," 248–51.

47. "What Pope Francis Learned from Homeless Girl: 'Cry with the Suffering!'"

Catholic News Agency, January 17, 2015, available at http://www.catholicnewsagency.com/news /what-pope-francis-learned-from-homeless-girl-cry-with-the-suffering-19592/.

48. Lawrence B. Finer and Rubina Hussain, "Unintended Pregnancy and Unsafe Abortion in the Philippines: Context and Consequences," Guttmacher Institute, August 2013, available at https://www.guttmacher.org/report/unintended-pregnancy-and-unsafe -abortion-philippines-context-and-consequences.

49. Stephen Vincent, "Filipino Church Vows Continued Opposition to 'Reproductive Health' Bill," *National Catholic Register,* December 20, 2012, available at https://www.ncregister .com/daily-news/filipino-church-vows-continued-opposition-to-reproductive-health-bill.

50. Sonia Narang, "Catholic Leaders Battle against Free Birth Control in the Philip- pines," *Public Radio International,* January 22, 2015, available at http://www.pri.org/stories /2015-01-22/catholic-leaders-battle-against-free-birth-control-philippines.

51. See Gerard O'Connell, "'*Amoris Laetitia*' Represents an Organic Development of Doc- trine, 'Not a Rupture,'" *America,* April 8, 2016, available at https://www.americamagazine.org /faith/2016/04/08/amoris-laetitia-represents-organic-development-doctrine-not-rupture.

52. See Michael G. Lawler and Todd A. Salzman, "*Amoris Laetitia*: Has Anything Changed?" *Asian Horizons* 11 (2017): 62–74.

CHAPTER FOUR

Ecclesiological Tensions in the *ERD*

We now turn our attention to ecclesiological tensions in the *ERD*. The first tension is between the hierarchical model of Church reflected in the *ERD*, with its insistent emphasis on the bishop's authority, "approved authors," and the lack of consideration or integration of the *sensus fidelium*, and the communion model embraced by the Second Vatican Council and Pope Francis. The second tension is ecclesiological *scotosis* of the impact of the sex-abuse crisis on the authority, credibility, and authenticity of bishops individually and collectively, a crisis that is neither acknowledged nor recognized in the revised *ERD*. We consider the first ecclesiological tension in this chapter and the second one in chapter 6.

HIERARCHICAL AND COMMUNION MODELS OF CHURCH

Prior to the Second Vatican Council in the 1960s, one approach to Catholic theology dominated all others. That approach was neo-scholastic and sought to produce timeless theological norms for a timeless Church, systematically stating theological positions, logically explicating them, and tenaciously defending them against all adversaries. The problem with this approach in the twentieth century turned out to be that it was not historically and therefore not theologically systematic enough. It could not stand as the official theology of a Church that, far from being timeless, came to be recognized as thoroughly time conditioned.

It could not stand in the light of the fundamental Christian norm that is sacred scripture, interpreted, as the Second Vatican Council taught, according to "what meaning the sacred writer intended to express and actually expressed in particular circumstances as he used contemporary literary forms *in accordance with the situation of his own time and culture*" (*Dei Verbum*, 11, emphasis added). It could not stand in the light of the riches of the fathers of the Church, East and West, also using literary forms in accordance with the situation of their own times and cultures. It could not stand in the light of a vital ecumenical movement that valued open and honest dialogue between Christians East and West and between Christians and non-Christians. Pope Francis recently described that dialogue as largely listening. "Keep an open mind," he advises. "Don't get bogged down in your own limited ideas and opinions, but be prepared to change or expand them. The combination of two different ways of thinking can lead to a synthesis that enriches both. The unity that Christians seek is not uniformity but a 'unity in diversity'" (*AL*, 139). Good advice, not only for Catholics in general but also for Catholic health care professionals and bishops in particular. For the followers of Christ in post-Holocaust Europe, in the postcolonial third world, in postmodern America, the twentieth century demanded a serious and honest "scrutinizing of the signs of the times and interpreting them in the light of the gospel" (*GS*, 4). In the Catholic Church, that scrutinizing was canonized by the Second Vatican Council and it led to the rejection of neo-scholasticism.

In preparation for a discussion on the nature of the Church at the Second Vatican Council in 1962, a theological commission prepared a draft document on the Church which, not surprisingly, was neo-scholastic in tone and content. It was arranged in four illuminating chapters, the "Nature of the Church," "Hierarchy in the Church," "Laity in the Church," and "States of Perfection in the Church," and there could be no doubt about its teaching. The Church is a hierarchical, almost monarchical institution ruled by consecrated bishops, with the bishop of Rome, the pope, as its supreme head. Authority in the Church belongs to popes and bishops; laity have no authority. Their job is to obey their bishops and the pope—to pray, pay, and obey as was commonly said at the time. When this preparatory document came to the council for discussion, it was roundly rejected by the council's bishops as a way to speak of Church in the twentieth century and returned to the preparatory commission to be reworked, not just cosmetically but at root, to bring it into line with Pope John XXIII's call for the *aggiornamento*, or updating of doctrinal language. It was suggestively rearranged in eight chapters, only three of which in their conciliar sequence need detain us here: "The Mystery of the Church," "The People of God," and "The Hierarchical Nature of the Church." It was overwhelmingly approved at the council's third session in November 1964 as *Lumen Gentium*, the Magna Carta of any subsequent reflection on, teaching about, and behavior of the post-conciliar Catholic Church. The revised *ERD* reads as if its composers never heard of that momentous document.

Dominican Yves Congar describes the transition from the council's preparatory document to *Lumen Gentium* as a transition from the priority of "organizational structures and hierarchical positions" to "the priority and even the primacy of grace."[1] We wholeheartedly endorse the truth in that description but still prefer a different one. The transition is from a juridical model that sees Church as hierarchical structure and institution to a theological model that sees it as graced communion and mystery to be plumbed in the never-ending search for a fuller Catholic truth. It is a transition from an exclusive focus on hierarchical office and authority to a focus on co-responsibility and synodality for belief and service. The rearrangement of the four neo-scholastic chapters of the preparatory document into the final eight, and especially the emphasis intended by placing the chapters on mystery and people of God before the one on Church hierarchy, provide ample evidence of the council's conviction that the Church is primarily a mysterious communion of believers with one another and with God in Christ before it is a hierarchical institution. Theologically interpersonal communion is prior to hierarchical institution, and that is as true in Catholic health care as in any other area of Church life.

The fundamental Catholic meaning of communion designates the communion of all the people of God with God in Christ and his Spirit, hence their common participation in Christian goods. The Church is first communion with God the creator, who created women and men for participation in divine communion (*LG*, 2); with the Son, who was sent "to establish peace or communion between sinful human beings [and God], as well as to fashion them into a fraternal communion" (*AG*, 3); and the Holy Spirit, who unites the Church in "a communion of fellowship and service" (*LG*, 4). It is second the fruit of communion with God, a communion in history of women and men with one another. An official note from the council in November 1964 explains that the model of Church as communion is not new but "an idea which was held in high honor in the ancient Church."[2] In his exhortation on the laity, *On the Lay Faithful*, Pope John Paul II characterizes the communion that is the Church as "the incorporation of Christians into the life of Christ, and the communication of that life of charity to the entire body of the faithful."[3]

The opening section of this chapter has one purpose: to make clear that two models of Church functioned and continue to function in the Catholic Church, a hierarchical model and a communion model, and that the Second Vatican Council determined that the communion model is primary and the hierarchical model secondary. A major theological tension in the *ERD* is its preference for the hierarchical model. It insistently highlights the authority of the local bishop in Catholic health care because of his ecclesiastical office, not his competence: "The ultimate responsibility for interpreting and applying of the Directives rests with the diocesan Bishop" (*ERD*, 25). He "exercises responsibilities that are rooted in his office [not competence] as pastor, teacher, and priest." In the absence of any determination by the magisterium, he is the one to determine "approved authors" for guidance in moral questions (*ERD*, 7). This is clearly a hierarchical approach not in line with the communion model that is the approved contemporary Catholic model of Church. The tension is not just that it is a hierarchical approach but that it completely ignores the implications of the communion model and its fellowship of service. This is nowhere more obvious in the document than in its suggested use of approved authors.

BISHOPS AND APPROVED AUTHORS

Some forty years ago, Archbishop Joseph Bernardin wrote on the relationship between the magisterium and theologians, recommending that two extremes be avoided. On the one hand, there cannot be any imperialism in which the magisterium co-opts theological scholarship as a mere mouthpiece for defending and propagating its teachings.[4] On the other hand, there cannot be secessionism between the magisterium and theologians that would grant theologians absolute autonomy and freedom from accountability. Instead, Bernardin proposes that in defining the relationship between magisterium and theologians, "it is essential to keep before us a reasonably clear and unambiguous notion of complementarity, particularly complementarity in the work of arriving at magisterial teaching."[5] He made no attempt, however, either to specify that notion of complementarity or to explain how it would be exercised. In this chapter, we attempt to do both, specifically with respect to Catholic health care.

Charisms are gifts of the Spirit intended for the building up of the communion Church, the body of Christ. Saint Paul teaches that spiritual gifts are given to each member of the body of Christ "for the common good" (1 Cor. 12:7) and lists a number of charisms (1 Cor. 12:8–11, 28–30). These and other texts have led many to conclude that ministry in Paul's churches was charismatic. The letters to Timothy, however, give a different account of ministry and the charisms associated with it. Ministry became more institutionalized and dominated by officeholders in the Church called *presbyteroi* (priests) and *episkopoi* (bishops), and charisms became more identified with those officeholders. In Timothy's church, the Corinthian ministry of those gifted with charisms appears to have been superseded by ministry exercised by presbyters and bishops. The legitimacy of their ministry is indicated not to any charisms they enjoy but simply by their being officeholders in the church. The real bearers of the Spirit to the Church, it appears, are now officeholders. This development marks the beginnings of a significant shift in the perception of ecclesiastical ministry and the charisms associated with it, and this shift created tensions throughout Christian history between charismatics and Church officeholders who seek to control their charisms.

After the Council of Trent in the sixteenth century, which seemed to understand the complementarity of the scholarship of theologians and the authority of bishops, the role of theologians changed from being consultants for, and collaborators with, bishops in teaching to being explainers and defenders of Church teaching already decided authoritatively by bishops. The term *magisterium* came to describe hierarchical officeholders and their teaching function. From being a servant of the truth, the hierarchical Church became a possessor and teacher of the truth, and ecclesiology became concerned almost exclusively with institutional factors in the Church. These factors concentrated on the institutional authority of hierarchical officeholders to the detriment of the scholarly authority of theologians. Pope Pius XII's statement in his 1950 encyclical *Humani Generis* regarding the task of theologians clearly sums up this development: "It belongs to them to point out how the doctrine of the living teaching authority [of officeholders] is to be found either explicitly or implicitly in the scriptures and tradition."[6] This is the same approach to Church authority found in the *ERD* with its insistence on the unchallenged role of the local bishop and of theological authors approved by him.

Fourteen passages in the documents of the Second Vatican Council include the terms *charisma* or *charismatic*, but their inclusion was not without tension. *Lumen Gentium* initially juxtaposes two kinds of gifts, hierarchical and charismatic (*LG*, 7), as if they are of a different nature, but later eases this tension, describing charisms as special gifts that the Spirit of God distributes among the faithful of every rank, making them "fit and ready to undertake the various tasks or offices advantageous for the renewal and upbuilding of the Church" (*LG*, 12). The council affirmed charism as a Spirit-given capacity and willingness for some kind of service that contributes to the renewal and upbuilding of the Church, but it struggled with the tension between the charisms gifted to all the faithful in the Church and the charisms gifted only to hierarchical officeholders. The *ERD* struggles with this same tension.

In 1996 the Vatican Congregation for the Doctrine of the Faith issued *Instruction on the Ecclesial Vocation of the Theologian*. What the *Instruction* includes in the theologian's charism, an emphasis on catechesis, and excludes, reference to any theological activity other than catechesis, makes it easy to conclude that it identifies the theologian's charism with catechesis. However, there is, we suggest, an important distinction between catechesis and theology that should always be maintained: "Catechesis is an education in the faith . . . which includes especially the teaching of Christian doctrine imparted . . . with a view to initiating the hearers into the fullness of Christian life" (*CCC*, 5). Though the theologian's task can certainly include catechesis, it is also more than catechesis. Theologians are scholars who employ scholarly principles and methods not only to communicate truths of the faith but also to explore those truths and new ways of articulating or formulating them, especially in the rapidly developing area of health care. Theologians have a double mediating function in the Church between the magisterium and the faithful. A first mediation comes before magisterial pronouncements; it requires theologians to do the preparatory work to get a sense of the questions, issues, and concerns of the faithful. The magisterium relies on this theological work to address any concerns in its pronouncements. A second mediation comes after magisterial pronouncements; it requires theologians to interpret and explain those pronouncements for the faithful in terms that are culturally, intellectually, and developmentally appropriate. The *Instruction*'s emphasis is clearly on this second mediation when it teaches that "the theologian is officially charged with the task of presenting and illustrating the doctrine of the faith in its integrity and with full accuracy."[7] Such a charge is clearly part of the theologian's vocation, but it does not exhaust the vocation that always includes the first mediation, the work of coming to a sense of the theological questions and their doctrinal and moral answers.

If bishops rely only on "the guidance of approved authors" (*ERD*, 7), often referred to as "safe theologians," for consultation in the first and second mediations—those who subscribe to official Church theology and function as theological apologists for it—other theological voices come to be silenced and ignored. Theologians who are unapproved authors and considered unsafe, whose scholarship leads to theological positions different from the bishop and his approved authors, are discounted in the consultative process. Including the ideas of only safe and excluding the ideas of unsafe theologians cuts like a two-edged sword. One edge permits the magisterium to claim that a doctrinal or ethical or health care pronouncement has been made with theological consultation and the agreement of theologians. The other edge sometimes provokes a critical theological response from those who have not been consulted, which earns them the unfair label of "dissenters." Determining whether or not a pronouncement communicates the faith of the whole people of God is settled in advance by a group of approved theologians, leaving those excluded from the consultative process with no other option but to be scholarly critical post-factum. There is, for instance, serious theological debate in the Church among professional Catholic ethicists over both beginning- and end-of-life issues, but Catholics would never know of those debates by reading the *ERD*, which echoes only official magisterial opinions as if they were the opinions of the whole competent communion Church.

This situation serves well no segment of the Church, neither magisterium nor theologians nor the entire body of the faithful. For the magisterium, it creates polarization between itself and the body of the faithful who massively disagree, for instance, with pronouncements about beginning-of-life issues and theologians who articulate this disagreement and formulate arguments that uphold it and challenge magisterial teachings. Their reflections are necessarily limited to either affirming magisterial pronouncements to be approved authors or critiquing them as not reflecting the beliefs of the vast majority of the communion Church, which leads to their being unfairly dubbed dissenters and unapproved authors. Many theologians are forced into the unfair and inaccurate classification of dissenters because they have been deprived of a consultative voice that might temper both the formulation of doctrinal and moral pronouncements and subsequent scholarly criticism of them. Basing magisterial pronouncements on the arguments of only those who hold a single Roman theology oversimplifies the complexity of a doctrinal or moral issue, especially in health care ethics, that would be better clarified by open scholarly, theological debate. This oversimplification sometimes results in magisterial pronouncements that rely more on ideology than compelling theological evidence and open and honest dialogue and consultation with the entire body of the faithful, the synodality Pope Francis proposes. Such an approach damages both the credibility of the bishops and the faithful's real understanding of highly complex Catholic truth.

Polarization also permeates the theological community. By consulting only with safe theologians, the magisterium implicitly endorses one school of theology over others and provides sanction for that school's work. This results in doctrinal and moral issues being settled by a claim of authority rather than by theological debate, which creates and perpetuates a vicious cycle among theologians. The magisterium issues pronouncements that rely on safe theologians; those safe theologians, buoyed by these pronouncements, cite them in the scholarly literature to justify their position and to attack theologians who disagree with them; and this inevitably, and incorrectly, leads to the labeling of these latter theologians as "dissenters," which leads to their further exclusion from every official consultation. There is evidence of this in the USCCB's recent document on racism, "Open Wide Our Hearts," which failed to consult with two of the leading theologians on race in the United States because of their controversial writings on women in the Church and sexual ethics. Narrowly defining the mediation of theologians as one of explaining and defending magisterial pronouncements forces "unsafe" theologians to serve not as consultants for but critics of magisterial pronouncements.

The lack of broad theological consultation can be damaging also to the entire body of the faithful, who detect a tension between the magisterium and a majority of Catholic theologians. These tensions are frequently aired by both magisterium and theologians in the media, and they often escalate into outright hostility, as in the Phoenix case. In this hostile climate of charge and counter-charge, complex issues are too often inaccurately or unfairly presented, serving neither side well and leading to suspicion, distrust, and cynicism among the faithful. Many lay theologians, who are contextually well placed to articulate lay issues and concerns, are not consulted, so magisterial pronouncements can appear detached from the lived reality of the lay faithful. This is noticeably true for health care in the *ERD*, as it is also true for sexual and women's issues.

There is another consideration: the demographics of theologians have evolved. Up until the Second Vatican Council, almost all theologians were clerics who taught primarily in seminaries; since the council, theology has become largely a lay profession exercised predominantly by lay women and men in Catholic and non-Catholic colleges and universities. This changed demographic has introduced voices into the theological conversation, especially women's and third-world voices, which have never before been heard in the conversation. These new voices challenge the traditional, male, hierarchical, Eurocentric voices that have historically dominated Catholic doctrinal and moral debates and demand that the magisterium take seriously the full scope of theological positions that exist in the communion Church (*LG*, 37). *Gaudium et Spes* expresses this judgment clearly and beyond doubt: "With the help of the Holy Spirit, it is the task of the *entire People of God*, especially pastors and theologians, to hear, distinguish, and interpret the many voices of our age, and to judge them in the light of the divine word." In this way, it adds, "revealed truth can always be more deeply penetrated, better understood, and set forth to greater advantage" (*GS*, 44, emphasis added). Pope Francis reflects this ecclesiology with his emphasis on synodality in both *Amoris Laetitia* and the Amazon Synod. The experiences of the entire people of God, of lay faithful, lay theologians, and especially of shamefully ignored lay women, reflect a Spirit-breath that requires communal, dialogical discernment to decide whether it confirms or challenges magisterial pronouncements. This is as true in Catholic health care as it is in university theology. Many contemporary lay Catholics are as competent as, and sometimes more competent than, diocesan bishops, not only in medical but also in doctrinal and pastoral issues.

The discipline of theology has also evolved. In the past, professional theological discourse took place in two contexts, between theologians and between professors and students. One of the most far-reaching changes effected by the Second Vatican Council was the empowerment of lay women and men to become more active in the Church, and with this increased activity, theology now has a third context, which may be described as an open public forum in the Church. Given their easy internet access to magisterial documents, theological magazines, and scholarly journals, laity are becoming ever more theologically educated, and theologians are now more in dialogue with the laity and speaking with and for them in teaching and writing. The community of Catholic theologians now has a responsibility to listen to contemporary educated Catholics' need for ethical understanding and action, and each individual theologian must accept her or his share of that collective responsibility, in ethical issues in Catholic health care as in all other ethical issues. The use of only approved authors seriously interferes with and curtails that responsibility.

An open forum, in health care issues as in others, will provide for competent lay women and men who share through baptism Christ's charisms of priest, prophet, and king (*LG,* 10–13) their right to be active in a teaching-learning Church. We recall here the judgment of consummate Church historian John Henry Cardinal Newman about the influence of the laity during the Arian controversy in the early Church. It was not the bishops, he judges, who saved the Church from the heresy of Arianism, for "the body of Bishops failed in their confession of faith," but the laity, who were "preeminent in faith, zeal, courage, and constancy." It was "mainly by the faithful people that paganism was overthrown."[8] We cannot help but believe that judgment is as true today in the era of rampant clerical abuse of all kinds as it was in the fourth-century era of Arianism. The demonstrated failure of many bishops points to and opens the way for a more adult and more dialogical Church that gives a genuine voice to the entire body of the faithful. Such an adult and dialogical Church, we believe, is adumbrated in Paul's extension of charisms beyond Church offices to individual believers for the upbuilding of the Church. It is also supported by a central teaching of the Second Vatican Council: "The body of the faithful as a whole, anointed as they are by the Holy One . . . cannot err in matters of belief" (*LG,* 12).

The responsibility of theologians as listeners to and teachers of the whole Church comes with the caveat that they must always be in dialogue with the whole communion Church—laity, other theologians, and office holders—as they seek to discern what theologically is and ought to be taught and done in new circumstances. The *Instruction's* implicit identification of theology as catechesis is incomplete, for theologians are called to serve the communion Church also through scientific investigation and exploration. They must always exercise their vocation guided by the virtues of prudence and caution in both their discernment of controversial theological and ethical issues and their presentation of them to the communion Church. It is essential, however, to the whole Church that they be free to exercise their vocation in the service of the Church as it pursues a deeper understanding and better formulation of doctrinal and moral teaching. The magisterium, on its part, must allow more open discussion and dialogue involving the whole communion Church—lay women and men, theologians, and hierarchy—without threat of disciplinary or punitive action, and must be patient in debates on controversial issues and slow to close such debates prematurely. That moral debates have been settled in the circumstances of the nineteenth and twentieth centuries is no guarantee that they remain settled in the new challenges of the twenty-first century, among which the *ERD* mentions "changes in religious orders and congregations, the increased involvement of lay men and women, a heightened awareness of the Church's social role in the world, and developments in moral theology since the Second Vatican Council" (*ERD*, 4). The tone of the *Instruction* neither evinces nor encourages the patience required from all groups in the Church, and neither does the revised *ERD* with respect to health care issues. We must look elsewhere for a model of the dialogue grounded in the "unity of charity" that the *Instruction on the Ecclesial Vocation of the Theologian* proposes.[9]

BISHOPS, DIALOGUE, AND THE *ERD*

The *ERD* frequently references the "diocesan Bishop," who the context reveals is the bishop of the diocese in which a Catholic health care facility is located. The bishop has oversight over the Catholic health care facility (*ERD*, 7) and oversight over appointments to the pastoral care staff of the facility (*ERD*, 12), over appropriate medical ethics standards in the facility (*ERD*, 15), and over the Catholic identity of and the adherence to Catholic teaching in the facility, especially when there is collaboration between Catholic and non-Catholic health care facilities (*ERD*, 25). There are some 3,042 Catholic health care facilities in the United States, ranging from trauma centers to hospitals to continuing care facilities, and these facilities employ some 739,500 full-time and part-time employees.[10] Catholic health care is a huge nationwide ministry, and occasionally there is a debate between responsible bishops over the interpretation and application of the *ERD*. The question for this section is how those debates ought to be approached and settled. The answer, we propose, is via a dialogue in charity, which we must explain before we proceed.

One of the implicit objectives of this commentary is to stimulate dialogue between all the health care members of the communion Church, but especially between theologians, approved and non-approved, and the magisterium. Pope Francis explains the necessity of such dialogue: "Keep an open mind. Don't get bogged down in your own limited ideas and opinions but be prepared to change or expand them. The combination of two different ways of thinking can lead to a synthesis that enriches both." He further explains that the unity we seek in the communion Church "is not uniformity but a unity in diversity" (*AL*, 139). While acknowledging that "the Church cannot furnish a ready answer to every moral dilemma" (*ERD*, 7), what the magisterial writers of the revised *ERD* and their approved theologians have given us is precisely traditional answers and health care uniformity in some ethically contested issues. These issues would be better synthesized in an open dialogue involving all the competent health care members of the communion Church. Pope John Paul II teaches that dialogue is rooted in the nature and dignity of the human person. It "is an indispensable step along the path towards human self-realization, the self-realization of each individual and of every human community. It involves the human subject in his or her entirety."[11] We agree that every dialogue must involve each participant in the dialogue. Each must attend carefully to the data emerging in the dialogue, which in health care ethics includes the selection, interpretation, prioritization, and integration of the four sources of ethical knowledge; must analyze the data intelligently; come to understand it; and formulate that understanding in mutually understandable concepts. Each must then judge the truth or falsity, certainty or probability, of his or her understanding. It is only after this judgment that any true knowledge is achieved in the dialogue. After the passing of judgment, the final step is to consider possible courses of action, evaluate them, make a decision about which course of action to follow, and then translate that decision into a course of action. The participants in any dialogue, including the dialogue about contested health care issues, must be equal partners, with none being privileged over any others, for it is only on the basis of this equality that any person in the dialogue may reach intellectual and perhaps also moral and religious conversion.

We are wide open to a health care dialogue in this commentary, and we highly recommend it. We must be, given the different theological and moral perspectives involved in health care, which we treat later in this chapter. We are like two men at a third-story window getting only a restricted third-story perspective on the landscape outside the window, and we must be open to the complementation of perspectives provided by people at sixth-, ninth-, and twenty-first-story windows. In traditional Catholic theological parlance, therefore, we situate this commentary in the category of *quaestio disputata*, the disputed question, so beloved of the medieval scholastics. The scholastic master had three tasks: *lectio*, or commentary on the Bible; *disputatio*, or teaching by objection and response to a theme; and *praedicatio*, or proclamation of the theological word. Peter Cantor speaks for all of them when he argues that "it is after the *lectio* of scripture and after the examination of the doubtful points thanks to the *disputatio*, and not before, that we must preach."[12] It is important for the reader to be aware that this commentary is *lectio* and *disputatio* before it is theological and pastoral *praedicatio*.

Internal Dialogue: *Sensus Fidei*

This commentary engages in two dialogues: one internal, the other external. The first dialogue is internal to theology and the Church. It asks what a two-thousand-year tradition has said and still has to say theologically and ethically about human anthropology, including its relevance for health care and how that ancient tradition is to be mediated to, appropriated by, and transmitted onward in and by the contemporary Church. The young Joseph Ratzinger, later to be Pope Benedict XVI, informs us why that internal dialogue must be pursued. "Not everything that exists in the Church," he argues, "must for that reason be also a legitimate tradition; in other words, not every tradition that arises in the Church is a true celebration of the mystery of Christ. There is a distorting, as well as a legitimate tradition and consequently tradition must not be considered only affirmatively but also critically."[13] In this commentary we accept Ratzinger's judgment as true for Catholic health care issues and consider them not only affirmatively but also critically.

Three matters are crucial to both internal dialogue and the critical consideration Ratzinger demands: the nature of Christian theology, the origin of Christian sacred scripture, and the nature of the Church, which claims its origin in the scriptures and seeks to mediate their meanings to each new Christian generation. The nature of the Church is, we believe, the most pressing of these three because how one conceives Church will determine how one conceives the functioning of another theological reality that is central to both the internal dialogue and to Catholic health care, namely, what is called theologically *sensus fidei*, "the instinctive capacity of the whole Church to recognize the infallibility of the Spirit's truth."[14]

Before we consider *sensus fidei*, however, we add another word about theology and theologians. Catholic theology prior to the Second Vatican Council was largely ahistorical, which explains its evident lack of creativity. One of the achievements of theologians schooled by the Second Vatican Council is to point the way beyond this ahistorical theology to a historically conscious, critical theology. Some still lament that some contemporary Catholic theology continues to live in a world that is passed and no longer exists, but we have chosen to ignore lament and move forward along the way limned by the Second Vatican Council, a theology that has implications for Catholic health care.

That perspective, the importance of which we have already explained in chapter 1 as perspectivism, is an important category in contemporary Catholic philosophy and theology and is an easily understood term with an easily understood everyday meaning. It can denote the outer limit of my physical vision, such as the line at which the earth and the sky appear to meet. Experience shows that physical perspective is not immovably fixed; it moves as I move, either receding in front of me or encroaching behind me. My perspective is determined by my physical position and, in turn, determines what I can and cannot physically see. Objects beyond my perspective I cannot, for the moment, see. Within my perspective lie objects I can see. My physical perspective provides an apt analogy for my personal perspective of knowledge. What lies within my personal perspective is, to a greater or lesser degree, an object of interest and of knowledge to me: I can be attentive to it, come to understand it, make a judgment about its truth, make an action-decision about it. What lies outside my personal perspective lies outside the range of my interest and knowledge.

There is both a similarity and a difference between my physical and personal perspectives. My physical perspective is determined by my physical position; my personal perspective is determined by my social position. There is, however, a difference. My physical perspective is determined by my physical position in my environment. I have no control over it other than to move my position. My personal environment is determined by my past socialization and my understanding and embrace of it; it constitutes both the condition and the limitation of my understanding and knowledge and of any possible development of either. My physical perspective is a given, simply because of where I physically stand; my personal perspective is a socially constructed position that can yield different cognitive perspectives that can be different and opposed. An understanding, a judgment, and a decision for action that is perceived as true in one perspective will be unintelligible and false in another perspective. Such is the situation with different bishops with different perspectives interpreting and applying the directives of the *ERD*. How are their different interpretations and applications to be reconciled and brought to a reconciled unity? As I have the freedom to move within a physical perspective to achieve a new perspective, so I have the freedom to move to a new personal perspective. Tutored by Canadian theologian Bernard Lonergan, we call the movement from one perspective to another conversion.

Lonergan judges that conversion, emphasized generally in Catholic ethical teaching and specifically in the recent Amazon Synod, is the movement from one perspective to another and that it may be intellectual, moral, or religious.

Intellectual conversion is "the elimination of an exceedingly stubborn and mis-
leading myth concerning reality, objectivity, and knowledge. The myth is that
knowing is like looking, that objectivity is seeing what is out there to be seen
and not seeing what is not there."[15] This myth confuses the physical world
of sensation—the sum of what is experientially seen, heard, touched, tasted,
smelled—with the world mediated by meaning, which is a world known not by
the act of seeing or any other sensation alone but by the cognitive process of
sensation, understanding, and judgment. Knowing is not simply seeing, hearing, touching, tasting, smelling; it is sensing, understanding, and judging. Until
knowers reach the judgment that their understanding is true or false, there is
no true knowledge. The myth that is to be clarified and eliminated has many
possible consequences. It can lead to naive realism, thinking that the world of
meaning can be known simply by looking at it, thinking that I achieve true
knowledge simply by looking at and learning what Saint Paul or Aquinas or
John Paul II said and wrote. Once intellectually converted from this prevalent
myth, I come to understand that what Paul or Aquinas or John Paul II wrote is
only a first step in the process of my coming to know, to be followed by my own
understanding and judgment, not only of what was said but also, and especially,
of what is true. The *ERD* is very much under the influence of the myth that
knowing is like hearing, citing from past scriptural and magisterial statements
with little or no analysis of their continuing relevance to the contemporary
human and health care situations (*ERD*, 4).

Besides intellectual conversion, there is also moral and religious conversion.
Following the judgment that attains truth comes the decision about what to do
about the truth. Moral conversion "changes the criterion of one's decisions and
choices from satisfactions to values."[16] Moral conversion involves progressively
understanding the present situation, exposing and eradicating both individual
and social bias, constantly evaluating my preferred values, paying attention to
criticism and protest, and listening to others. Neither one instance of moral
conversion nor one moral decision leads to moral perfection, for after one
conversion there remains the possibility of either yet another conversion or a re-
lapse, and after moral decision there is still required moral action. Conversion is
not to be conceived as a once-in-a-lifetime moment but as an ongoing process.

Religious conversion "is being grasped by ultimate concern. It is other-
worldly falling in love. It is total and permanent self-surrender without conditions, qualifications, reservations."[17] It is, in Christian terms, falling in love with
God. Human love always releases humans to transcend themselves; think of the
love of parents for their children, the love between friends, the love between
lovers. Love demands self-examination and commitment, dissolves biases and
polarities, and enables conversion from one perspective to another. When we

are in love, especially in love with God, a new perspective emerges and takes over, and the love of God becomes the all-controlling perspective. Intellectually, morally, religiously converted bishops; theologians, both those who enjoy episcopal approval and those who do not; and all believing Catholics are intellectually, morally, and religiously competent to engage in dialogue about Catholic health care, and their voices should be heard. In the most recent revision of the *ERD*, they are not heard. That is a great detriment to the analysis and directives, and it shows.

Perspective and conversion have much to do with what is called *sensus fidei* in the communion Church. *Sensus fidei* is a spiritual charism of discernment, possessed by the whole Church, which recognizes and receives a teaching as Catholic truth and, therefore, to be believed. It has biblical root in Paul's exhortation to the Philippians to "have this [common] mind among yourselves, which is yours in Christ Jesus" (Phil. 2:5). It has modern validation in the Second Vatican Council, which taught that the doctrine of the Catholic Church is preserved in *all* the faithful, laity and hierarchy together. "The body of the faithful *as a whole,* anointed as they are by the Holy One (1 John 2:20, 27), cannot err in matters of belief [that is, they are infallible]. Thanks to a supernatural sense of the faith [*sensus fidei*] which characterizes the people *as a whole,* it manifests this unerring quality when, 'from the bishops to the last of the faithful,' it manifests its universal agreement in matters of faith and morals" (*LG*, 12). Catholic doctrine enshrines this belief in its teaching that the Spirit is gifted to the whole Church. That teaching makes sense only in a Church that is believed to be and is lived as a communion instituted by Christ, constituted by the Spirit of Christ, "a new brotherly community composed of all those who receive him in faith and in love" (*GS*, 32). It is from and for such a Church, and particularly for everyone in health care ministry in that Church, that this commentary is written to invite conversion and an ongoing communional search for intellectual, moral, and religious truth.

Internal Dialogue: The Bishops

This search for truth through conversion, dialogue, and discernment between bishops and the *sensus fidei* is also a search for truth between the bishops of dioceses spanned by single Catholic health care institutions. Part 6 of the revised 2018 *ERD*, "Collaborative Arrangements with Other Health Care Organizations and Providers," is the main revised section and addresses collaboration between Catholic and non-Catholic health care institutions guided by the principles governing cooperation, which we address in detail in chapter 6. A central point of the revisions is to assert and strengthen the authority of the local bishop to make authoritative decisions regarding the nature of such collaborations and to interpret and apply the principles guiding those collaborations. Here, we focus on the dialogue and collaboration *between bishops* when a health care provider, such as Common Spirit Health, has entered into a collaborative relationship with a Catholic provider, spans several dioceses, and is under the authority of several bishops. How are disagreements between bishops on the interpretation and application of the *ERD* in general, or the interpretation and application of the principles governing cooperation in particular, to be negotiated canonically and ethically? We respond to these questions in light of canon law and the process proposed by Pope Francis, synodality, which impacts internal and external dialogue in Catholic health care institutions.

The *ERD* and the Authority of the Bishop

Since the Church's beginning, there have been disagreements between bishops and leaders in the Church. Paul confronts Cephas (Peter) in Antioch on what Paul perceives to be his hypocritical treatment of Jews and Gentiles regarding circumcision and dietary laws, opposing Peter "to his face because he clearly was wrong" (Gal. 2:11–14). Such disagreements between leaders in the Church persist. Cardinals Raymond Burke, Carlo Caffarra, Walter Brandmüller, and Joachim Meisner recently published a letter, technically called a *dubia*, accusing Pope Francis of fostering confusion among the faithful in *Amoris Laetitia*.[18] The cardinals' *dubia* highlights the current polarization in both the US and worldwide Catholic Church between both traditionalist and progressive bishops and traditionalist and progressive theologians. This polarization in the United States extends to how different bishops understand, interpret, and apply the *ERD*.

The *ERD* asserts the authority of a diocesan bishop to interpret and apply the *ERD*, to assess any collaborative relationship between Catholic and non-Catholic health care institutions in his diocese, and to approve any such collaborative relationship (dir. 69). It also affirms his responsibility to discern if there is any "wrongful cooperation" in such relationships (dir. 67). In the process of discerning collaboration, the bishop is to consider "not only the circumstances in his local diocese but also the regional and national implications of his decision" (dir. 67). In cases where a health care system spans several dioceses, the diocesan bishop that has jurisdiction over the system's headquarters has a special role "to initiate a collaboration with the diocesan Bishops of the dioceses affected by the collaborative arrangement" (dir. 69). The *ERD* implicitly recognizes the potential for disagreements among bishops on the nature of this collaboration. "The Bishops involved in this collaboration," it decrees, "should make every effort to reach consensus" on the collaborative relationship, but it provides no guidelines for resolving potential conflicts on the interpretation and application of the *ERD*. We must look elsewhere for such guidelines.

CANON LAW AND THE AUTHORITY OF THE BISHOP

Lumen Gentium (27) decrees that the Bishop is the vicar of Christ in his diocese, and both the 1983 Code of Canon Law, frequently called the final document of the Second Vatican Council, and the *Catechism* confirm this decree: "Though each Bishop is the lawful pastor only of the portion of the flock entrusted to his care, as a legitimate successor of the apostles he is, by divine institution and precept, responsible with the other Bishops for the apostolic mission of the Church."[19] The bishops' pastoral roles are as "teachers of doctrine, priests of sacred worship, and ministers of governance." Their ministry of governance is legislative, judicial, and executive.[20] Episcopal consecration establishes a basic equality among all bishops; they possess "ordinary, proper, and immediate power to govern their dioceses except in those areas reserved to supreme Church authority [the pope] or another higher level of Church government [a bishops' conference]."[21] Unfortunately, the 1983 Code of Canon Law left ambiguous the precise relationship between canons guiding the particular Church and the bishop governing that Church and canons guiding the intermediate level of Church government that is a bishops' conference.[22] This canonical ambiguity is not addressed or resolved in the *ERD*.

The *ERD* is a document issued by an intermediate level of Church authority, the USCCB, and it serves as an authoritative guide for individual bishops to oversee Catholic health care institutions in their respective dioceses. The *ERD*, however, does not provide any guidelines for resolving conflicts that may emerge between bishops when there is collaboration between Catholic and non-Catholic health care institutions spanning several dioceses, and it is left up to individual bishops to resolve, without any road map, conflict arising from the collaboration. Both the canonical and *ERD* guidelines allow a great deal of latitude for interpretation and application of the *ERD* as long as there is no explicit violation of Catholic doctrine. Such an approach creates ambiguity when different bishops may have different perspectives on what is or is not an acceptable interpretation of the *ERD* and its rules for cooperation between Catholic and non-Catholic health care institutions.

In line with canon law, the *ERD* grants autonomy and independence to individual bishops. This arrangement, however, has been revealed as deeply troubling in the age of uncovered clerical sexual abuse when some individual bishops, acting autonomously and independently, covered up the sexual abuse, and other bishops did not challenge them until the extent of the abuse and cover-up became public knowledge in 2002. It is hard to believe that, given the overwhelming public and theological disagreement with Bishop Olmsted and his interpretation and application of the *ERD* in the case of Sister Margaret McBride and Saint Joseph's Hospital and Medical Center, no other bishop spoke out publicly to challenge his decisions. There seems to be a fear among many bishops to publicly challenge an individual bishop's decisions lest, in return, they be publicly challenged as well. This reticence among US bishops to challenge one another has reinforced a hierarchical and clerical model of Church, has created a dysfunctional Church, and has damaged bishops' credibility and moral authority. Given the scandals of the Phoenix case and the sex-abuse crisis, the *ERD*'s lack of guidelines for resolving disagreements between bishops results in a missed opportunity for peaceful resolution of conflicts that may further damage the bishops' voice on moral issues.

In addition to the *ERD*'s failure to provide specific guidelines for resolving conflicts between bishops, we call attention to two further specific points in the teaching ministry of the bishop that bear on the process of interpreting and applying the *ERD*. First, in exercising his teaching ministry, a bishop is called to promote doctrinal integrity while allowing a certain degree of freedom to the faithful, especially to faithful experts in a specific area, to clarify the mysteries of faith, which includes ethical teaching surrounding health care.[23] A noteworthy development in the 1983 Code of Canon Law is its direction to the bishop that he is to exhort the faithful "to exercise the apostolate according to each one's condition and ability and is to exhort them to participate in and assist the various works of the apostolate according to the needs of place and time."[24] This communion ecclesiology highlights the importance of the *sensus fidei* in the life of the Church and the need for bishops to consult the faithful in discerning doctrinal and moral integrity.

Second, the canonical mandate to involve a broad cross-section of the people of God in the pursuit of the Church's mission can most aptly be realized through the process of synodality at the core of Pope Francis's papacy. As explained in chapter 3, synodality implies all members of the Church—laity, minor clerics, and bishops—journeying together and receiving input from one another toward the discernment of the will of God for the Church and the path the Church must follow to live according to that will. Such synodality, which demands "dialogue in charity," was exemplified in the two synods on the family to which Pope Francis's *Amoris Laetitia* is a response. That synodality, unfortunately, has not been embraced by the USCCB in its revision of the *ERD*, nor is it mentioned in the *ERD* as a process for reaching consensus in disagreements between bishops that might arise in collaborative relationships between Catholic and non-Catholic health care institutions. This is a missed opportunity.

In a speech a week before the November 2019 meeting of the USCCB, a speech that theologian Massimo Faggioli labeled the US equivalent of Pope Francis's 2017 "magna carta" speech on synodality, Bishop Robert McElroy of San Diego declared, "It is my reluctant conclusion that the Church in the United States is now adrift on many levels and that a fundamental moment of renewal is needed. A synodal pathway would be an opportunity to set that type of renewal in motion. . . . The great danger is that our ecclesial life is becoming like our political life—polarized, distorted, and tribal. That is why a deep and broad process of synodal dialogue within the Catholic community in the United States could empower an alternative pathway forward."[25] His words on polarization were verified at the USCCB meeting, but his prophetic message of synodality to heal the polarization of the bishops went unheeded.[26] The USCCB seems to be locked into the polarization that both Pope Francis and Bishop McElroy warn against. This polarization is evidenced in the *ERD*'s repeated reference to "approved authors" who are to be invited to serve as consultants for the bishop when interpreting and applying the *ERD*.

Pope Francis, Bishop McElroy, and the International Theological Commission all propose synodality as a way to move the Church beyond polarization by inviting all the faithful, those who agree and those who disagree, to the table of dialogue to move the Church forward from stagnant polarization. The ITC suggests that "the criterion according to which 'unity prevails over conflict' is of particular value in conducting a dialogue, managing different opinions and experiences and learning 'a style of constructing history, a vital field where conflicts, tensions and opposites can reach a pluriform unity which generates new life,' making it possible to 'build communion amid disagreement.'" Dialogue, it continues, "offers the opportunity to acquire new perspectives and points of view in order to shed light on the solution of the matter in question."[27] To build the recommended "communion amid disagreement" in a polarized Church, all Church members—laity, minor clerics, bishops, approved and unapproved authors, even the disaffected—should be invited to the table of synodality and dialogue. Without such synodality and dialogue, we assert, the polarization infecting the Church can only persist.

External Dialogue

The second dialogue necessarily involved in this commentary is a dialogue external to theology and to Church. It takes place between Catholic theology, ethics, and values and the different theology, ethics, and values held by groups with which Catholic health care institutions cooperate. The bishop in whose diocese such cooperation takes place "has the ultimate responsibility to assess whether collaborative arrangements involving Catholic health care providers operating in his local Church involve wrongful cooperation, give scandal, or undermine the Church's witness" (dir. 67). We must say a word about scandal, though we address the principles governing cooperation, scandal, and witness in detail in chapter 6.

The *Catechism of the Catholic Church* defines *scandal* as "an attitude or behavior which leads another to do evil. . . . Scandal is a grave offense if by deed or omission another is deliberately led into a grave offense" (*CCC*, 2284). It further teaches that "anyone who uses the power at his disposal in such a way that it leads others to do wrong becomes guilty of scandal and responsible for the evil that he has directly or indirectly encouraged" (*CCC*, 2287). The *ERD* cites this teaching (*ERD*, 30). The giving of scandal is a serious ethical issue and something to be avoided. What is not clear, however, is how claims of scandal are to be justified. Catholic health care workers should certainly lead by word and example, and they should be supportive of the teachings of the Catholic Church. Scandal, however, can depend on which teaching of the Catholic Church is emphasized. The *ERD* advances Catholic teaching on "actions that are intrinsically immoral, such as abortion, euthanasia, assisted suicide, and direct sterilization" (dir. 70), but nowhere does it focus on the Catholic teaching on the authority and inviolability of the responsibly informed conscience, which we deal with in the next chapter. Human dignity, the Second Vatican Council teaches, demands the right to follow one's conscience (*GS*, 16), and violating the consciences of health care workers or of cooperating non-Catholic institutions, thereby possibly justifying discrimination against them, might give scandal every bit as much as performing a direct sterilization. Scandal, in other words, lies in the eye of the beholder, and, we ask, which claim of scandal is justified in any complex health care ethical situation? The assertion that an action would cause scandal is precisely that, an assertion, not a theological or ethical argument. Like any other assertion of ethical right or wrong, it must be justified by sound ethical argument.

The *Catechism* teaches that "the Church's social teaching proposes principles for reflection; it provides criteria for judgment; it gives guidelines for action" (*CCC*, 2423). This trinity—principles for reflection, criteria for judgment, and guidelines for action—is underscored in John Paul II's *Sollicitudo Rei Socialis*. This approach to social morality, an authentically established part of the Catholic moral tradition in modern times, introduces a model of converted personal responsibility that underscores the responsibility of each person in the communion Church in any dialogue. John Paul II accentuates this Catholic perspective by explaining that, in its social teachings, the Church seeks "to guide people to respond, with the support of rational reflection and of the human sciences, to their vocation as responsible builders of earthly society" (*SRS*, 1). This teaching applies also to any dialogue in a Church that is communion seeking to responsibly build Catholic health care: Church teaching *guides*; responsible believers, drawing on Church guidance, their own experience, understanding, conscience, decisiveness, and the findings of the human sciences, *respond*. "Catholic health care should be marked," the *ERD* teaches, "by a spirit of mutual respect among caregivers" (dir. 2), and so should any internal or external dialogue about it. Dialogue about any issue, including health care, should always be characterized by personal freedom, not by unquestioned obedience to external authority consistently implied in the *ERD*.

The notion of responsibility introduces an important dimension of individual and communional freedom to the unnuanced notion of uncritical obedience. In social reality like cooperative health care, the magisterium does not pretend to pronounce on every last detail or to impose final decisions. It confesses that "it cannot furnish a ready answer to every moral dilemma" (*ERD*, 7), thereby leaving judgment, decision, and action to faithful and responsible consciences. Sociomoral principles are humanly constructed guidelines for attention, understanding, judgment, decision, and action, not moral imperatives drawn from divine, natural, or ecclesiastical law, and demanding uncritical obedience to God, nature, or the Church. John Paul adds what the Catholic tradition has always taken for granted. On the one hand, the Church's social teaching is "constant." On the other hand, "it is ever new, because it is subject to the necessary and opportune adaptations suggested by the changes in historical conditions and by the unceasing flow of the events which are the setting of the life of people and society" (*SRS*, 3). Principles remain constant. Judgments and actions, as history amply demonstrates, can change after responsible reflection on changed historical and social contexts and the ongoing flow of human events illuminated by the social sciences. Since this approach is authoritatively advanced in social morality, it should be employed in any decision about the morality of Catholic health care. Part of the proposal of this commentary is, under the guidance of authentic Catholic theological and moral principles and the illumination of the contemporary sciences, to refer questions about health care morality to the theologically, morally, and religiously converted informed conscience.

Christians in general, including approved and non-approved Catholic theologians and Catholic health care professionals, do not live in a comfortable ecclesiastical cocoon. They live in a real world with other human beings, many of whom appear to have decided that Christians have nothing to tell them about that world, about themselves in that world, or about Catholic health care in that world. Many of these other health care professionals have perspectives on the world and answers for the world's health care questions that differ from Catholic theological, moral, and religious perspectives and answers. That raises the unavoidable question of which perspective guides to truth, a question that in turn raises the question about a necessary external dialogue between Catholic and other perspectives. Individuals and the human world they inhabit are not two independent realities; they are realities that work in an ongoing dialectical and symbiotic interdependence. Human society, culture, perspective are human products that act back on their producers to conform and control them. The temptation of intellectually unconverted individuals, be they theologians or not, is always to assume that *our* way is the *right* way and *our* truth is the *real* truth. The sociology of knowledge scotches that unconverted approach.[28]

CONCLUSION

Human truth is always subject to a given perspective of meaning and is supported by a plausibility structure that derives from that perspective. Each perspective has its own accent of reality, its own cognitive style, its own consistency and compatibility, and outside of a given perspective it is difficult, if not impossible, to grasp the truth held within that perspective. That raises the specter of relativism, so disconcerting to many, including Pope Benedict XVI, who frequently refers to it as a root cause of the Church's problems. Relativism acknowledges that all human truth is inseparably bound to the historical perspective of the thinker and concludes that, therefore, all human truth is relative and unreliable. We do not accept that judgment. All human truth is, indeed, inseparably bound to the sociohistorical perspective of the thinker and is, therefore, *relational*, but that does not suggest it is unreliable. It suggests only that truth-within-perspective is partial truth in need of complementation by truths held in other perspectives. That suggestion is even truer, the Christian traditions universally teach, when it comes to human truth about God, whom "no one has ever seen" (John 1:18; cf. Ex. 33:20–24).

The God whom the communion Church believes in is always a transcendent mystery, always present to limited people but always beyond their intellectual grasp. Recognizing this Christian theme, the magisterium of the Catholic Church teaches that "the fullness of truth received in Jesus Christ does not give individual Christians the guarantee that they have grasped that truth fully. . . . Christians must be prepared to learn and to receive from and through others the positive values of their traditions. Through dialogue they may be moved to give up ingrained prejudices, to revise preconceived ideas, and even sometimes to allow the understanding of their faith to be purified."[29] Such should be the attitude of bishops and Catholic health care institutions when they enter into cooperation with non-Catholic health care institutions. Pope John Paul II approves. Dialogue, he teaches, "is rooted in the nature and dignity of the human person. . . . [It] is an indispensable step along the path towards human self-realization, the self-realization of each individual and of every human community. . . . It involves the human subject in his or her entirety."[30] It is in such synodal dialogue, we have suggested, that differences between bishops and between bishops and non-approved theologians in interpreting and applying the *ERD* will be resolved.

We make only one proviso: the dialogue about Catholic theological, ethical, and health care issues should include as far as possible every member of the communion Church; remember that "the body of the faithful as a whole, anointed as they are by the Holy One, cannot err in matters of belief. Thanks to a supernatural sense of the faith which characterizes the People [of God] as a whole, it manifests this unerring quality when, from the Bishops down to the last member of the laity, it shows universal agreement in matters of faith and morals" (*LG*, 12). The phrase contained in that conciliar statement of Catholic faith, "from the Bishops *down* to the last member of the laity," manifests a remnant of a hierarchical attitude in the bishops of the Second Vatican Council. Half a century later, that hierarchical attitude is still present in the revised *ERD*.

SUGGESTED READINGS

Bernardin, Joseph. "Magisterium and Theologians: Steps towards Dialogue." *Chicago Studies* 17, no. 2 (1978): 151–58.

Lonergan, Bernard J. F. *Method in Theology.* New York: Herder, 1973.

Newman, John Henry. *On Consulting the Faithful in Matters of Doctrine.* New York: Sheed and Ward, 1961.

Pontifical Council for Interreligious Dialogue. *Dialogue and Proclamation.* Vatican City: Typis Polyglottis Vaticanis, 1991.

Salzman, Todd A., and Michael G. Lawler. "Theologians and the Magisterium: A Proposal for a Complementarity of Charisms through Dialogue." *Horizons* 36 (2009): 7–31.

Thiel, John E. *Senses of Tradition: Continuity and Development in the Catholic Faith.* New York: Oxford University Press, 2000.

NOTES

1. Yves M. J. Congar, "The People of God," in *Vatican II: An Interfaith Appraisal*, ed. John H. Miller (Notre Dame, IN: University of Notre Dame Press, 1966), 197–207, at 199.

2. Walter M. Abbott, ed., *The Documents of Vatican II* (London: Chapman, 1966), 99.

3. Pope John Paul II, *Christifideles Laici*, 19.

4. The term the *magisterium* refers to both hierarchical officeholders and their teaching function in the Catholic Church.

5. Joseph Bernardin, "Magisterium and Theologians: Steps towards Dialogue," *Chicago Studies* 17, no. 2 (1978): 151–58, at 158.

6. Pope Pius XII, *Humani Generis*, 21.

7. Congregation for the Doctrine of the Faith, *Instruction on the Ecclesial Vocation of the Theologian* (Vatican City: Libreria Editrice Vaticana, 1996), 22.

8. John Henry Newman, *On Consulting the Faithful in Matters of Doctrine* (New York: Sheed and Ward, 1961), 10.

9. Congregation for the Doctrine of the Faith, *Instruction on the Ecclesial Vocation of the Theologian*, 26.

10. Catholic Health Association of the United States, *Incarnate Grace: Perspectives on the Ministry of Catholic Health Care* (Saint Louis, MO: Catholic Health Association of the United States, 2017), 3.

11. John Paul II, *Ut Unum Sint*, 28.

12. Peter Cantor, *Verbum Abrreviatum*, 1, *PL*, 205, 25.

13. Joseph Ratzinger, "The Transmission of Divine Revelation," in *Commentary on the Documents of Vatican II*, vol. 3, ed. Herbert Vorgrimler (New York: Herder and Herder, 1969), 181–92, at 185.

14. Thiel, *Senses of Tradition*, 47.

15. Bernard J. F. Lonergan, *Method in Theology* (New York: Herder, 1973), 238.

16. Lonergan, 240.

17. Lonergan, 240.

18. See Staff Reporter, "Full Text: Cardinals' Letter to Pope Francis on *Amoris Laetitia*," *Catholic Herald*, November 14, 2016, available at https://catholicherald.co.uk/full-text-cardinals-letter-to-pope-francis-on-amoris-laetitia/.

19. *CCC*, 1560; *Code of Canon Law*, c. 381.

20. Canon Law Society of America, *Codex Iuris Canonici* (Washington, DC: CLSA, 1983), Canons 375.1 and 391.1.

21. Thomas J. Green, "Title I: Particular Churches and the Authority Established in Them," in *The Code of Canon Law: A Text and Commentary*, ed. James A. Coriden, Thomas J. Green, and Donald E. Heintschel (New York: Paulist Press, 1985), 311–49, at 320, 314.

22. Green, 313.

23. Green, 315.

24. *Code of Canon Law*, c. 394.2.

25. Massimo Faggioli, "Adrift and Alone: The Bishops Meet, and Miss the Point," *Commonweal*, November 25, 2019, available at https://www.commonwealmagazine.org/adrift-alone; Bishop Robert McElroy, "Bishop McElroy: US Church Is Adrift, Synodality Can Renew It," *National Catholic Reporter*, November 7, 2019, available at https://www.ncronline.org/news/opinion/bishop-mcelroy-us-church-adrift-synodality-can-renew-it.

26. See Michael Sean Winters, "U.S. Bishops' Conference Clearly Divided between Team Francis, Culture Warriors," *National Catholic Reporter*, November 13, 2019, available at https://

www.ncronline.org/news/opinion/distinctly-catholic/us-Bishops-conference-clearly
-divided-between-team-francis-culture.

27. International Theological Commission, "Synodality in the Life and Mission of
the Church," March 2, 2018, 111, available at http://www.vatican.va/roman_curia/congre
gations/cfaith/cti_documents/rc_cti_20180302_sinodalita_en.html.

28. See Michael G. Lawler, *What Is and What Ought to Be: The Dialectic of Experience, Theology,
and Church* (New York: Continuum, 2005).

29. Pontifical Council for Interreligious Dialogue, *Dialogue and Proclamation* (Rome: Typis
Polyglottis Vaticanis, 1991), 49.

30. John Paul II, *Ut Unum Sint*, 28.

CHAPTER FIVE

Pastoral and Spiritual Care in the *ERD*

Part 2 of the *ERD* deals with "The Pastoral and Spiritual Responsibility of Catholic Health Care." It opens by grounding human dignity in a double characteristic, creation in the image of God (Gen. 1:26) at the beginning of life and destiny to share a life with God at the end of life. This double characteristic is shared by all human beings, and "Catholic health care has the responsibility to treat those in need in a way that respects" their shared dignity and destiny (*ERD*, 10). Pastoral care and spiritual care immediately cry out for definition so that we can know what we are talking about, and there is in the *ERD* a broad description of pastoral care. It includes "a listening presence [or invitation to dialogue], help in dealing with powerlessness, pain, and alienation; and assistance in recognizing and responding to God's will with greater joy and peace" (*ERD*, 10). There is no description of spiritual care.

In not-too-distant Catholic history, the word *spiritual* was reserved for monks and nuns who were striving to be religious by living both a rigorous lifestyle withdrawn from worldly experience and a disciplined prayer life at the heart of the Church. Fueled in part, but certainly not exclusively, by clerical sexual abuse and its scandalous cover-up by bishops, many Catholics now describe themselves as *not very religious* but deeply *spiritual*. If religion is in serious trouble, theologian Sandra Schneiders comments, "spirituality is in the ascendancy and the irony of this situation evokes puzzlement and anxiety in the religious establishment, scrutiny among theologians, and justification among those who have traded the religion of their past for the spirituality of their present."[1] The root of this postmodern Catholic spirituality is earthly and holistic human experience. Schneiders defines it as "the experience of conscious involvement in the project of life integration through self-transcendence toward the ultimate value one perceives. It is an effort to bring all of life together in an integrated synthesis of ongoing growth and development."[2]

Jungian psychiatrist David Tracey also emphasizes the centrality of individual experience in contemporary spirituality, pointing out that "today it is felt to be the living heart of the individual and the location of spirituality has shifted from tradition to experience." Experience, he continues, "has been elevated above tradition and spirituality has been elevated above religion." Spirituality in its contemporary garb, then, embraces the experience of every person as a whole, bodily, psychologically, socially, and religiously, and it embraces specifically the presence of God incarnate in the depth of that experience. Tracey believes that this contemporary spirituality can be accommodated by traditional religion, but only if it is "prepared to place experience before dogma and individual encounters with God before the rules and regulations of religion."[3] We agree, and this chapter seeks to illuminate the presence of God in the individual human experience of sickness.

SACRAMENT

The traditional Catholic way to make the incarnate God explicitly present is the way of sacrament, and the *ERD* insists that "provision for the sacraments is an especially important part of Catholic healthcare ministry" (dir. 12). It singles out the celebration of the sacraments of the Eucharist (dir. 12), penance (dir. 13), and anointing of the sick (dir. 15). Many Catholics, including many untrained pastoral ministers, do not fully grasp the Catholic theology of sacraments with the result that they look on them as mechanistic devices for making the hidden God present, but sacraments are far from mechanistic. They are prophetic symbols, modeled on Jesus the Christ, believed to be the incarnate symbol of God, in and by which the Catholic communion Church, the sacramental body of Christ, proclaims, makes real, and celebrates for believers the presence and action of God, which is called grace. A brief commentary on that definition will summarize and clarify that Catholic meaning of sacrament.

Since Augustine, it has been traditional to understand sacraments as signs of the presence of the hidden God. They are, however, not simple signs like a stop sign or a sale-price sign but a specialized kind of sign called symbol and, indeed, that specific kind of symbol called prophetic symbol. A prophetic symbol is an ordinary human action that on the physical level of reality has an ordinary meaning but that on the symbolic level of reality has quite another set of meanings. Water, for instance, on the physical level means cleansing, life, and

sometimes death. On the symbolic level, therefore, immersion in water is apt
to proclaim, make real, and celebrate in symbolic representation cleansing from
sin, death, and resurrection to new life, as it does in baptism. On the physical
level marriage means the contracted communion of two persons, along with
their mutual love, mutual caring, mutual service. On the symbolic level, therefore, it is apt to proclaim, make real, and celebrate the covenanted communion
of Christ and his Church, along with their mutual love, mutual caring, and
mutual service, as it does in the sacrament of Christian marriage.

A sacrament is a prophetic symbol, established by and modeled on Christ
the symbol of God. By being himself, on the physical level, a Jewish man who,
on the symbolic level, is believed by Christians to be the sacrament of God,
Jesus established patterns for sacramental reality. In its actions the Church follows these established patterns, and when it acts formally as the body of Christ,
as it does in the celebration of the Eucharist, its actions are the actions not just
of these gathered women and men but symbolically also of Christ. Such actions
of the Church, therefore, are themselves sacramental actions. On a physical
level, they appear to be ordinary, natural actions: immersion in water, anointing with oil, sharing a meal of bread and wine, uniting in a marriage, but on a
symbolic level, they are far from ordinary, natural actions. They are prophetic
symbolic actions, proclaiming, making real, and celebrating in symbolic reality,
respectively, the death and resurrection of Jesus and of believers, the presence
of the Spirit of God in believers, the presence of the crucified and risen Christ
in his sacramental body, the loving and indissoluble union between Christ and
his Church. To the extent that these prophetic symbolic actions are patterned
on Christ the incarnation or embodiment of God, we can rightly say that they
were established or instituted by him.

Though signs and symbols always have meaning, they do not always *effectively*
have meaning for every person. The flag of France means something quite different for French and Americans and so too does the flag of the United States.
The same is true of sacramental and prophetic symbols. A prophetic symbol
is always celebrated to proclaim the presence and action in the Church of God
and God's Christ, but whether it *effectively* proclaims, makes real, and celebrates
that presence for any given person depends on that person. The Catholic theological tradition requires the intentional action of a free person, who believes
in, trusts in, and accepts the presence of God mediated in this symbol. Only
when such a personal activity is brought to the symbol does the symbol become
an *effective* symbol for a person, and only then does it *effectively* proclaim, make
real, and celebrate the presence and the action in the Church of God in Christ.
The active faith of believers who share the faith of the Church transforms ordinary, natural actions into far-from-ordinary symbols and sacraments. This is

why the *ERD* decrees that "normally, the Sacrament [of anointing of the sick] is celebrated only when the sick person is fully conscious" and that it can be celebrated for the unconscious sick only "if there is reason to believe that they would have asked for the sacrament while in control of their faculties" (dir. 15). The celebration of any sacrament for an unconscious person is a decision not to be made lightly since it always runs the risk of the suspicion of mechanistic magic.

Every Catholic has learned in religious instruction that sacraments confer the grace they signify *ex opere operato*, a doctrine they interpret to mean that they confer grace automatically. Sacraments, however, do not confer grace automatically; they confer grace not because of the correct positing of some mechanistic action but because of the combined personal actions of God, God's Christ, and the believer actively participating in the action. It is God in Christ who effects grace, not an external sacrament, however precisely and validly executed, and it is a believer who either actively accepts that grace or inactively ignores it. Grace is something ultimately and uniquely personal and interpersonal. The personal character of grace demands an equally personal response, for personal connotes freedom, responsibility, active acceptance, not mechanistic automaticity. It is for this reason that unconscious sick persons should not be involved in the celebration of any sacrament. God in Christ always exists for humans as offered; he exists not only as offered but also as accepted only when humans freely, responsibly, and conscientiously accept him in faith. The personal faith, love, hope, and trust expressed in their free reception of a sacrament is precisely the behavior that permits actualization of the sacrament as an effective symbol. The work of God in Christ and the work of the believer come together for any effective sacrament. The teaching of the fifteenth-century Council of Florence stands unchanged: sacraments give grace to those who receive them worthily, and that is as true for sick Catholics as for healthy ones.

The basic sense of grace in the Catholic tradition is adumbrated in Saint John's teaching: "In this is love, not that we loved God, but that God first loved us" (1 John 4:10). In theological language, God giving Godself in love is called uncreated grace. The effect of this personal love, which transforms women and men and their world, is called created or sanctifying grace. Grace, therefore, has two traditional theological meanings: first, God self-giving in love, and, second, a transformation produced in those who believe. These two meanings are, of course, intimately related. God, who is uncreated grace, creates men and women and their world and offers Godself to them at their creation, which means that women and men live always and everywhere, even in sickness, in a radically graced world. Creation is the first grace, in which God creates humans, dwells in and with them as uncreated grace, and invites them into personal, loving, and

transforming, sanctifying grace. If this is so, if women and men live in a fundamentally graced world, what is the specific contribution of Christian sacraments to the living of a life of grace, a life of relationship with God? Uncreated
grace, the loving self-gift of God to all women and men, exists long prior to
any sacramental action. Every man and woman created by God is enveloped in
grace, for uncreated grace is God himself in his gracious love. Because of this
offered uncreated grace, history for every person is really a history of possible
grace and salvation, quite apart from any sacramental activity. Sacraments, however, the Catholic Church teaches, make that uncreated grace explicitly effective
for those who believe.

As with the man and woman who do not *effectively* recognize their mutual
love until they make love in some symbolic action—they hug, they kiss, they
share a special meal—neither do men and women recognize the presence of
the God who is grace until they make grace in some symbolic action. Though
sacraments are not the only ways to make grace, they are religiously established
Catholic ways to make grace. When believers engage in sacramental action, they
proclaim, make real, and celebrate in it not only the presence of grace offered
to them by God but also that grace personally accepted by them. The gracious
offer of God and the faithful acceptance of that offer by believers together, in
and through the prophetic and symbolic and sacramental action, make grace.
The grace that is made present is none other than God; only secondarily, and as
a consequence of God's presence and action, is it the justifying transformation
of believers that Catholics have learned to call sanctifying grace.

We have sought to explain that sacraments are prophetic symbols in the
Church, actions that on one level of reality are ordinary actions but on another
level are far from ordinary symbols that proclaim, make real, and celebrate in
representation the presence of God in Christ. We add one final insight into
sacrament and its specific connection to Catholic health care. It has been traditional to reserve the word *sacrament* for the seven ritual sacraments of the
Catholic Church: baptism, confirmation, reconciliation, Eucharist, matrimony,
holy orders, and anointing of the sick. In contemporary Catholic theology, the
meaning of the word has been extended. It is applied to Christ, who is said to
be the sacrament of God in human history. It is applied to the communion
Church, which is said to be the sacrament of Christ in human history. It is
applied to actions of the communion Church in human history, not only to
the actions that are the traditional seven sacraments but also to every action
of the communion Church and of its believing members that puts them in
touch with the presence of God in human experience. Theologian Karl Rahner
distinguishes the seven solemn ritual actions of the communion Church and
the everyday actions of the Church and its believing members as Sacrament

(uppercase) and sacrament (lowercase), respectively. When the actions of the communion Church, whether solemn ritual actions or everyday actions, are met with and interpreted by the faith of believers, those actions are transformed into sacraments of the presence and action of God in Christ in human history. When the caring action of a nurse or a physician toward a sick person in a Catholic or non-Catholic health care institution, therefore, is offered and met with faith and interpreted by the sick person as not only a medical action but also the symbolized action of God in Christ, then that caring action has been transformed into a lowercase sacrament of the action of God and Christ in human history. The experience of physical medical care has been elevated to the experience of the sacramental presence and action of God. That is how important Catholic health care is theologically, for both the health care professional who offers caring actions in faith and for the sick who in faith can transcend sickness to experience the sacramentalized presence of God.

This explanation of sacraments establishes God and Catholic believers and their experiential relationship as ultimately important, whether the believers are healthy or deathly sick. It lets sacraments be important as symbols of a divine-human relationship; it lets believers be as present to God in Christ as God in Christ is present to them. God and believers relate not exclusively in two or nine or even twenty-nine sacraments, but in uncountable symbolic, sacramental ways, not only within the Catholic communion but also outside it. Sacraments do not grace and save; only God in Christ graces and saves, but in and through sacraments. And God graces and saves all those people, Christian and non-Christian alike, who actively cooperate with God's saving grace. In the relationship between God in Christ and historical people, faith and sacramentally mediated presence is all there is; only in death will both faith and sacrament give way to possessing and being possessed. "For now we see in a mirror dimly," Paul writes to his Corinthians, "but then face to face. Now I see in part; then I shall understand fully, even as I have been fully understood" (1 Cor. 13:12).

The mystery of God in Christ and Christ in Church and its believing members illuminates every aspect of Catholic health care; divine love and grace actively and conscientiously offered and responded to by human love is its animating principle. We are arguing here that the compassion and care of Catholic health care professionals and the resultant personal and spiritual healing of sick patients is one more sacramental moment proclaiming, making real, and celebrating the presence and healing ministry of Jesus the Christ. This sacramental reality is the reason why, even though Bishop Olmsted incredibly removed from Saint Joseph's Hospital and Medical Center both the hospital's "Catholic" status and the Eucharist, it still remains a place of sacramental ministry and compassion where care is offered and received in faith. No action of any bishop can ever remove the sacramental and pastoral reality of Christ's presence in faith-filled health care.

Spiritual response to suffering is one more moment for looking into the interior, spiritual depth of experience and finding there both the God in Christ who is always there and the conviction that death is not a moment that separates us from that God but a wonderful moment that allows us to see no longer in a mirror dimly but face to face (*ERD*, 6). Catholic health care ministry must be a ministry to whole physical, relational, psychological, spiritual sick people, inviting them to plumb the depth of their experience and to find there the God who is eternally gracious in sickness and in health, even, perhaps especially, in the face of death that frequently terrifies even the firmest of believers.

CONSCIENCE

A foundational Catholic teaching, spiritually vital in both sickness and health, is sadly missing in the *ERD*, namely, Catholic teaching on conscience.[4] Pope Francis complains that we "find it hard to make room for the consciences of the faithful, who very often respond as best they can to the Gospel amid their limitations and are capable of carrying out their own discernment in complex situations." He insists that "we have been called to form consciences, not to replace them" (*AL*, 37). That is good advice for Catholic teachers at all levels. In the thirteenth century, Thomas Aquinas established the authority and inviolability of conscience: "Anyone upon whom the ecclesiastical authorities, in ignorance of the true facts, imposes a demand that offends against his clear conscience, should perish in excommunication rather than violate his conscience."[5] Seven hundred years later, the last century of which saw the rights of individual conscience essentially ignored in the Catholic Church, it continues to be ignored in the revised *ERD*: "Catholic health care does not offend the rights of individual conscience by refusing to provide or permit medical procedures that are judged morally wrong by the teaching authority of the Church" (*ERD*, 8). The Second Vatican Council's *Gaudium et Spes*, however, issued a clarion cry with respect to the authority of conscience: "Conscience is the most secret core and sanctuary of man. There he is alone with God whose voice echoes in his depth. In a wonderful manner conscience reveals that law which is fulfilled by love of God and neighbor" (*GS*, 16). The council's Decree on Religious Freedom went further to assert the inviolability of conscience: "In all his activity a man is bound to follow his conscience faithfully, in order that he may come to God for whom he was created. It follows that he is not to be forced to act contrary to his conscience. Nor, on the other hand, is he to be restrained from acting in accordance with his conscience, especially in matters religious" (*DH*, 3). This solemn and inviolable Catholic teaching is in effect in the sick as in the healthy and is a mandatory element in health care for every conscious patient and every health care professional. When faced with the loss of consciousness, patients may commit their judgments of conscience to a legally binding advance directive.

The word *conscience* denotes an act of practical judgment on a particular ethical issue commanding us to do this or not to do that. It comes at the end of a process of discernment, which is a process of experience, understanding, judgment, decision. To make a practical judgment of conscience involves gathering as much evidence as possible, consciously understanding and weighing the evidence and its implications, and finally making as honest a judgment as possible that this action must be done and that action must be avoided. Since this process ends with a judgment about what is good or evil, right or wrong, we call it an *ethical* process. Conscience, we insist, is not a law unto itself but must be as fully informed as possible to be right. That formation is precisely the process from gathering the necessary evidence, discerning the evidence, to making the practical judgment that this is what I must do in this situation.

Since conscience is a practical judgment that comes at the end of a deliberative process, it necessarily involves the virtue of prudence, by which "right reason is applied to action" (*ST*, II–II, q. 47, a. 5). Prudence is a *cardinal* virtue around which all other virtues pivot. No moral virtue, Aquinas argues, can be possessed without prudence, since it is proper to moral virtue to make a right choice (*ST*, I–II, q. 65, a. 1). Unfortunately, as human experience amply demonstrates, even the most prudential practical judgment can be in error. That raises the question of the erroneous conscience, so at this point we need to introduce some important distinctions. Moral theologians note that there are two poles in every moral judgment. One is a subjective pole, for it is always a free, rational human *subject* who makes a judgment; the other is an objective pole, since every judgment is made about some objective reality, giving alms to the poor, for instance, or choosing to forgo some painful clinical treatment. Subjects arrive at their judgments either by following the correct rational process or by somehow short-changing that process. In the first case, the subject arrives at a right ethical understanding and conscience judgment about the object; in the second case, the subject arrives at a wrong or erroneous understanding and conscience judgment about the object. If a decision to forgo some medical treatment follows a right understanding and judgment about the treatment and its effects on the patient, then conscience is also said to be right; if it follows an erroneous understanding and judgment of the treatment and its effects on the patient, then conscience is also said to be erroneous.

If the error of understanding and judgment can be ascribed to some fault, taking little trouble to find out what is the good in the situation, for instance, or negligent failure to gather the necessary evidence, to engage in the necessary discernment, to take the necessary advice, then the wrong understanding and the practical judgment of conscience flowing from it are both deemed to be culpable and cannot be ethically followed. If the error cannot be ascribed to some ethical fault, then both the understanding and the practical judgment of conscience flowing from it are deemed to be non-culpable and not only can but must be followed, even contrary to Church authority. Joseph Ratzinger, later Pope Benedict XVI, explains: "Over the Pope as the expression of the binding claim of ecclesiastical authority there still stands one's own conscience, which must be obeyed before all else, if necessary, even against the requirement of ecclesiastical authority. Conscience confronts [the individual] with a supreme and ultimate tribunal, and one which in the last resort is beyond the claim of external social groups, even of the official Church."[6] There is one final distinction to be added here. The morality of an action is largely controlled by the subject's motive. A good motive, forgoing some surgical treatment *because* of the debilitating expense to one's family, is a moral thing to do. A bad motive, forgoing the surgery treatment *because* the surgeon is black, for example, is a bad, racist motive and will result in an immoral action.

A decision of right conscience is a complex process. It is an *individual* process but far from an *individualistic* process. The Latin word *con-scientia* literally means "knowledge together," perhaps better rendered in English as "knowing together." It suggests what human experience universally demonstrates, namely, that being freed from the prison of one's individual self into communion with others is a surer way to come to right ethical truth and judgment of what one ought to do or not do. This communion basis of the search for Christian truth and ethical action builds a sure safeguard against both an isolating egoism and a subjective relativism that negates all universal truth. The communion dimension of consciences has been part of the Christian tradition since Saint Paul, who clearly believed in the inviolability and primacy of conscience (1 Cor. 10:25–27; 2 Cor. 1:12; 4:2; Rom. 14:13–23). It is within this communion of consciences that Church authority functions, not guaranteeing conscience (past errors preclude that simplistic claim) but informing it to a right practical judgment. We are instructed here by Saint John Henry Cardinal Newman's famous comment to the Duke of Norfolk: "If I am obliged to bring religion into after-dinner toasts (which indeed does not seem the right thing), I shall drink to the Pope if you please, still to conscience first and to the Pope afterwards."[7]

The Catholic faithful, the International Theological Commission teaches, "have an instinct for the truth of the Gospel, which enables them to recognize and endorse authentic Christian doctrine and practice, and to reject what is false." It continues: "Banishing the Catholic caricature of an active hierarchy and a passive laity," so prevalent in the *ERD*'s emphasis on the authority of the local bishop in Catholic health care, "and in particular the notion of a strict separation between the teaching Church and the learning Church, the Council taught that all the baptized participate in their own proper way in the three offices of Christ as prophet, priest, and king. In particular it taught that Christ fulfills his prophetic office not only by means of the hierarchy but also via the laity."[8] The attainment of moral truth in the Catholic tradition, therefore, involves a dialogical process in the communion Church between the "bishops down to the last member of the laity" and, when that process has been conscientiously completed, even the last member of the laity is finally "alone with God whose voice echoes in his depths" (*GS*, 16) and must make that practical judgment of conscience that this is what I must believe or not believe, do or not do. Back to Newman's dictum, and to Aquinas's and Ratzinger's: first, conscience and, afterward, the pope and the Church.

Having made a practical judgment and decision of conscience, no Catholic is "to be forced to act in a manner contrary to his conscience. Nor . . . is he to be restrained from acting in accordance with his conscience, especially in matters religious" (*DH*, 3) and also medical. This instruction applies to every sick conscious patient and to the struggling family of the unconscious patient. The *Catechism of the Catholic Church* places the Church's teaching beyond doubt: Catholics have "the right to act in conscience and in freedom so as personally to make moral decisions" (*CCC*, 1782). A well-informed, and therefore well-formed, conscience is the Catholic way to choosing the true and the good in both health and sickness. That Catholic teaching ought to be included in every ethical situation, including every health care situation, but it is noticeably missing in the revised *ERD*.

PLURALISM AND POLARIZATION

An obvious characteristic of the contemporary Catholic Church is the doctrinal and moral pluralism exhibited by its members. Some are absolutely opposed to abortion; others argue that abortion is morally acceptable in certain circumstances. Some argue that for the permanently vegetative state patient artificial nutrition and hydration is a natural means of preserving life, not a medical act, and should be considered in principle as an ordinary and proportionate means of preserving life (*ERD*, dir. 58). Others argue that there should be a presumption in favor of providing ANH to all PVS patients only as long as its benefits outweigh burdens for patients and their families. Such pluralism has created divisive polarization in the Church, the creation of two poles of opinion that is proving destructive in the Church, as it is also in political society. Such polarization, we suggest, is not needed in the face of plural opinions; they can easily be explained by the metaethical theory of perspectivism, which is to be carefully distinguished from relativism. Relativism rejects all objective, universal truth; perspectivism acknowledges objective, universal truth but insists that humans can attain such truth only partially, though adequately and reliably. Whatever truth humans can attain is never to be considered the only possible correct truth but a truth that is always in need of further clarification and development. The International Theological Commission's "Theology Today" advances ethical pluralism created by partial truths as an essential criterion of Catholic theology.[9]

Pope John Paul II writes of the centrality of perspective, noting that "in order to be able to grasp the object of an act which specifies that act morally, it is necessary to place oneself in *the perspective of the acting person*" (*VS*, 78; emphasis added). Perspective is easy to understand via the visual analogy of a man in a multistory building. He looks out a first-story window and sees what that window allows him to see; he then looks out a tenth-story window and a twenty-fifth-story window and sees the more that those windows allow him to see. What he sees outside the three windows, though different and clearly partial to the extent that our viewer can see only what each window allows him to see, put into partial but adequate and reliable focus what truly lies outside each window. When you look out a first-story window, you see what truly lies outside the window; when you look out a twenty-fifth story window, you see what truly lies outside the window. Perspective is also what accounts for different moral judgments. Seeing and judging from different perspectives accounts for the different judgments on the morality or immorality of abortion and of removing ANH from a PVS patient.

In the introduction, when speaking of metaethics, we introduced Bernard Lonergan's theory of perspectivism with respect to human knowledge and truth. It applies to our present question of ethical pluralism in the Catholic Church in that different definitions of human dignity, for instance, and of various moral norms derived from those different definitions, are rooted in different perspectives on morality. Just as his perspectives from windows on three stories in his building give the man access to different, partial, but adequately and reliably true views of what truly lies outside his building, so also the approach to questions about morality from two intellectual perspectives will lead him to two partial but possibly true answers to questions about morality and the principles, norms, directives, and judgments that facilitate or frustrate its attainment. The perspectives he uses to look at morality limit what he can see and judge about both it and the moral principles that control ethical judgments. This metaethical, perspectival approach confronts every charge of relativism and shows it is not sustainable. Writing on the nature of historical knowledge, Lonergan puts the foregoing in stark philosophical language: "Where relativism has lost hope about the attainment of truth, perspectivism stresses the complexity of what the historian is writing about and, as well, the specific difference of historical from mathematical, scientific and philosophic knowledge."[10] In plain language, looking from different mathematical, philosophical, medical, and theological perspectives will lead to different conclusions about human dignity and the implications of those conclusions for ethical decision and action. Relativism, we repeat, concludes to the falsity of a judgment; perspectivism concludes to its partial but adequate and reliable truth.

A non-ethical analogy will help to explain the perspectivist model we are highlighting. In 2015 "the dress" phenomenon, in which a photograph where a dress appears as either black and blue or white and gold, depending on the viewer, flooded social media. The phenomenon demonstrates differences in physiological perceptions of color that is a research interest of neuroscientists. While we do not want to examine in depth here what neuroscience research demonstrates, the dress phenomenon illustrates an important point about how human beings know. When the brain is confronted with "profound uncertainty," such as the uncertainty of color, it fills in gaps in its knowledge by making assumptions based on past experiences of sensory perception, lighting, and color.[11] On these bases, individuals judge that the dress is either black and blue or white and gold. It is incorrect to declare that one judgment is right and the other judgment is wrong since, for any given individual, sensory perception, lighting, color, and historical experience are what inform that judgment and ground the partial truth of that judgment for that individual. What all can agree on is that it is a picture of a colored dress. This "dress color phenomenon" offers an analogical parallel to perspectivism that accounts for both universal agreement and individual differences. People can have the same object or ethical situation before them, the dress or a pregnant woman with severe, life-threatening pulmonary hypertension, and come to different conclusions about the nature of the object or ethical situation depending on their physiology or ethical perspectives, respectively. They can also agree on universals: this is a dress, not a car; some medical experiments on human beings are ethical and some are always unethical. Common human experience would predict that, if both our man at a lower window and our health care ethicist were to ascend to a higher level, they would each get a different but no less partial, adequate, and reliable view.

Every human judgment of truth, including every judgment of ethical truth in health care situations, is a limited judgment based on limited data and understanding. "So far from resting on knowledge of the universe, [a judgment] is to the effect that, no matter what the rest of the universe may prove to be, at least this is so," and an ethical judgment of a well-informed conscience is to the effect that, no matter what the rest of the universe may prove to be, at least this action is to be done and that action is to be avoided.[12] It is precisely the necessarily limited nature of human understandings and judgments that leads to perspectivism, not as to a source of falsity but as to a source of partial but adequate and reliable truth. If this is so, and we agree with John Paul II that it is, then perspectival, partial, adequate truth is not a reason for polarization or division in the Catholic Church. It is rather a reason for the dialogue of charity advanced by Pope Francis. "Don't get bogged down in your own *limited* ideas and opinions," he advises, "but be prepared to change or expand them. The combination of *two different ways of thinking* can lead to a synthesis that enriches both." The unity we seek, he continues, "is not uniformity, but a 'unity in diversity' or 'reconciled diversity'" (*AL*, 139). Polarization in ethical issues relating to health care, or in any moral or doctrinal issue, is contrary to the Catholic way, for it endangers the common good to which "Catholic health care seeks to contribute" (*ERD*, 8).

Not every moral question has a definitive answer, and the *ERD* confesses that "the Church cannot furnish a ready answer to every moral dilemma" (*ERD*, 9). What is the proper response, then, to moral and doctrinal pluralism in the Church? The definitive answer to that question is that dialogue in charity and unity in diversity is the Catholic way. Pope Francis insists that mercy, which is preceded by empathy, the capacity to feel what another person is feeling, must always be pastorally active when judging ethical situations (*EG*, 44). Empathy and mercy, therefore, must also be active in the plural opinions about ethical action in every health care situation.

In summary, there is broad metaethical agreement within Catholic moral theology. First, it accepts metaethical objectivism; there *are* objective, universal definitions of human dignity and objective judgments of health care moral issues, even if they are as yet only partially but adequately and reliably grasped. Second, it defines the ethical terms *good* and *right* in relation to an objective definition of human dignity. Third, given different perspectives, different Catholic moralists can and sometimes do disagree on both the definition of universal human dignity and the formulation and justification of objective norms that facilitate or frustrate its attainment, including in health care issues. Fourth, perspectivism, which recognizes the inherent limitations of human knowledge, helps to account for the different definitions of human dignity and the different formulations and justifications of objective norms that facilitate or frustrate its attainment in every ethical issue, including health care ethical issues. Fifth, the variability that arises from perspectivism is an essential part of an objectivism that recognizes universals; the good is objectively defined as human dignity. Different objective definitions of human dignity and of the ethical norms flowing from it are not indications of relativism that denies universal truth but the unavoidable outcome of viewing ethical questions from different perspectives. Sixth, polarization in ethical issues, including ethical issues in health care, is not the Catholic response to pluralism; dialogue in charity is the Catholic response.

DISCERNMENT

Conscience is a practical judgment that this action rather than any other is the ethical action to be done in this situation. That definition leaves a critical question: How is that practical judgment to be arrived at? Pope Francis hints at a Catholic answer in the citation we offered at the beginning of this chapter: the faithful "are capable of carrying out their own *discernment* in complex situations." Discernment, which is a thoroughly *theo-logical activity*, is the Catholic way to reach a decision of conscience. We are not saying that non-Catholics have no need to or cannot discern, for they too can and must discern their situations and reach practical conscience judgments for their actions to be ethical. When we say that for Catholics discernment is a *theo-logical* activity, we are saying that it is both a spiritual gift and skill to uncover the presence and activity of God in every experience and decision in their lives. When Catholics discern, they are seeking two things. They are seeking, first, the presence and action of God in their lives, especially what God is calling them to do in a particular situation. They are seeking, second, the action they must do in this situation to be aligned with God's will and, therefore, to be ethical. We say it is a gift because it is given to us at our creation by our creator God; we say it is a skill because the gift can and must be honed and developed by practice. As gift and skill, discernment is not unlike riding a bicycle. First, my parents give me a gift of a bicycle for my ninth birthday, and then, by constant practice, I develop the skill to ride the bicycle with ease. Catholic health care professionals need the skill of discernment in crucial health care issues.

When Catholics discern, we said, the first thing they seek to discern is the presence and action of God in their lives. Spiritual writer Mark McIntosh distinguishes five moments in the process of discernment, the first of which is the discernment of the presence and action of God in our lives.[13] Trust in that God, a theological virtue, provides the foundation for Catholic discernment and for the ethical action that is its outcome. This first moment involves ridding our minds of all worldly distraction and ways of thinking, ridding it of what Sigmund Freud called the *superego*, prescriptions and proscriptions for doing this or not doing that from authoritarian figures in my childhood, parents, teachers, priests, so that I would be deemed a good boy or a good Catholic. Saint Paul recommended this clearance of mind to his Roman converts: "Do not be conformed to this world, but be transformed by the renewing of your minds, so that you may discern the will of God" (Rom. 12:2). The second moment in the process of discernment is the discerning of good and evil desires and biases that distort our perceptions and make our discernment of the presence and action of God and of our ultimate practical judgment of conscience more difficult. Again Saint Paul instructs us: "The works of the flesh are obvious: fornication, impurity, licentiousness, idolatry, sorcery, enmities, strife, quarrels, dissensions, carousing" (Gal. 5:19–26). We can easily add our own lists of evils, greed, idolatry of money, refusing to share our goods with the poor, racial hatred, and, today, fear of immigrants.

The third moment of discernment is a moment of practical wisdom that demands maturity, both human and Christian. It demands the experience-based human maturity to intuitively reach the most ethical action in a situation. It demands the Christian maturity to recognize not only the presence and action of God in our experiences but also the ethical action toward which God is impelling us in a particular situation. This recognition of both the presence and action of God and the action toward which God is leading us opens onto the fourth moment of discernment, the moment when I recognize that this action in this situation is God's will for me. This recognition in turn leads us into a broader vision of Christian truth, a larger perspective from which to view our actions, a twentieth- rather than a third-floor window to see beyond the ethical action toward which we are now impelled. The fifth and final moment of discernment is the moment we judge that this action rather than that one is God's will for us in this specific situation and we freely decide to do it. This final moment is the moment of the judgment of conscience, and following that practical judgment into action is the moment we act ethically.

Exercising personal autonomy in any situation, including any health care situation, and making one's own decision based on discerned factors is never easy, for we all carry with us Freud's *superego*: parental, clerical, and cultural authoritarian hangovers from childhood, the deeply rooted, authoritative proscriptions and prescriptions commanding us to do this and not do that in order to be a good child or a good Catholic. The superego is frequently confused with conscience, but there is a vast difference between them. The superego is the remnant of childhood training that was intended to guide our social and religious behavior when we were as yet unable to make our own proper ethical choices. That childhood training, however, took place at a time when our dependence on some adult authority was necessary, but that dependence on the authority of others for our ethical decisions was never intended to be permanent. It was always intended to give way to the autonomous practical judgments of our informed consciences when we had reached the personal and cognitive maturity to be autonomous. Saint Paul's instruction to the Corinthians accurately describes the difference between the superego and conscience: "When I was a child, I spoke like a child, I thought like a child, I reasoned like a child; when I became a man, I gave up childish ways" (1 Cor. 13:11). Among the childish ways adults must give up is the superego. That is not to say that all childhood instructions are to be overthrown in our maturity. As mature Catholic adults we still should not tell a lie, should not steal our sister's things, should be nice to that old grouch Mr. O'Driscoll who refused to return every ball that found its way into his backyard, but not because our mother or Father Burke said so. No, we should not tell a lie or steal or swear at Mr. O'Driscoll, because in our maturity we are able to discern the practical conscience judgment that this is what we must do and not do to be a mature and ethical human being and Catholic.

The age-old question of free will, so crucial in judging ethical responsibility, arises at this point. Free will implies the ability to choose freely one thing rather than another and is the sine qua non of morality. Without free will, we would not have the ability to choose our actions freely and would consequently have no moral responsibility for them. Neuroscience, the science of the human brain, raises serious questions about free will. Many neurological studies show an association between the process of willing and increased energy in the brain's frontal lobes. "Right here," researchers Jeffrey Schwartz and Sharon Begley assert, "you can say while pointing to the bright spots on the PET scan, volition originates."[14] The critical question, of course, is which comes first, the increased frontal lobe energy or the volitional act? If the brain energy comes first, then it can be argued that our actions are determined by brain energy; if the volitional act comes first, then we exercise free will. As a result of his extensive experiments with obsessive-compulsive disorder patients, whom he found can be trained to choose and to have thoughts other than their obsessive-compulsive ones, Schwartz argues that humans do have free will and are responsible for their actions. He explains his conclusion by arguing for what he calls mental force, "a physical force generated by mental effort," which is "the physical expression of will . . . [and] physically efficacious."[15] Mental force enables humans to make a free choice of this action or that. There is no determinism.

Schwartz traces the cause of this mental force to the outcome of "effortful attention." He marvels that at the end of the nineteenth century, without any of the modern neuroscientific research tools, psychologist William James had already reached the same conclusion. "Effort of attention," James wrote, "is thus the essential phenomenon of will." Schwartz responds, "The causal efficacy of will is a higher-level manifestation of the causal efficacy of attention. To focus attention on one idea, on one possible course of action among the many bubbling up inchoate in our consciousness, is precisely what we mean by volition."[16] Free will acts through attention that focuses on and makes predominant one thought or one action out of the many that are possible. Attention, however, is only the first part of what *will* means. There is a second part, consent to the reality that is attended to. Schwartz found in his experiments that "for the stroke victim, the OCD [obsessive-compulsive disorder] patient, and the depressive, intense effort is required to bring about the requisite refocusing of attention."[17] Intense effort, we suggest, is required also for everyone seeking to discern the will of God in every ethical situation, including every health care situation. Freely chosen effortful attention generates the mental force that is required for any discernment and ethical choice. Personal *intention*, so crucial in ethics, is made causally efficacious through personal effortful *attention*.

We consider finally another personal and social factor for those seeking discernment and conscientious ethical action, one we have referred to frequently in the preceding pages of this commentary, namely, human experience. Catholic ethicist Joseph Selling declares that *Gaudium et Spes* "stands as a milestone in the evolution of Roman Catholic moral theology."[18] It states that "there are a number of particularly urgent needs characterizing the present age, needs which go to the roots of the human race. To a consideration of these in the light of the Gospel and of *human experience*, the Council would now direct the attention of all" (*GS*, 46, emphasis added). The paragraph significantly shifts method in Catholic ethics by rooting them not only in scripture and Catholic tradition but also in human experience. A legitimate question, however, immediately arises: whose experience is to be used in the formulation of a Christian morality?

We emphasize that experience is never a stand-alone source of moral theology; it is only one factor to be considered in discerning a moral judgment and action. "My experience" alone is never a source. Moral authority in the Catholic Church is granted only to "our experience," to communion-Church experience, and only in constructive dialogue with scripture, tradition, and reason and science. There is little to be gained from simply encountering the world in which we live; many people have many such encounters and learn little from them. The experience we speak of here intends "the human capacity to encounter the surrounding world consciously, to observe it, be affected by it, and to learn from it."[19] It is of the essence of such experience that it is never raw, neutral encounter with the world; it is always interpreted by both individuals and communities in specific sociohistorical perspectives. It may, therefore, be interpreted differently by "me," by "you," by "us," and by "them." For genuine human experience as we have defined it, the dialectic is necessarily a "dialectic of reason *and* experience" and never a dialectic controlled by either reason or experience alone. In a church that is a communion of believers in God in Christ, the resolution of different understandings of experience to arrive at shared moral truth requires an open spirit of collegiality and a respectful dialogue of charity. Such dialogue must occur in the communion of believers, some of whom are laity, some of whom are theologians, and some of whom are clerics, all of whom acquire knowledge through practice or action, that is, through experience. The *ERD* subverts this communional interpretation of experience by its persistent reference to the authority of the local bishop and his "approved authors" advisers (*ERD*, 7, 25, dir. 67).

Contemporary Catholic moralists espouse an inductive methodology that begins with human experience and seek a common experience on which to found and formulate ethical norms. Lisa Sowle Cahill articulates well the relationship between human experience and ethical norms: "The essential point to emphasize for an ethics which begins with, and remains respectful of, differences in experience, while not giving up the possibility of normative ethics, is that the 'shared' is not achieved beyond or over against [experience], but rather in and through it."[20] Human realities do not always conform to some preformed ideal, not even to some preformed Church ideal, so ethically right choices will often depend more on prudent, practical adaptation of the ideal to the experiential reality than on the ideal itself. The challenge is to carefully discern what constitutes authentic experience that may revise the definition of human dignity and norms and directives that facilitate attaining it and what constitutes inauthentic experience that must be judged by an established definition of human dignity and its corresponding norms or directives. Catholic ethicists consider four sources of ethical teaching to discern that definition and to formulate and justify those norms and directives for health care issues: scripture, tradition, experience, and science. They do not consider only the "body of moral principles [that] has emerged that expresses the Church's teaching on medical and moral matters" (*ERD*, 4), for changed experience and circumstances might demand changed moral principles, directives, and actions. When the music changes, so also does the dance.

ACCESS TO HEALTH CARE

As we noted in our introduction, Christians believe that Jesus of Nazareth is God incarnate in the world, that he is "the way, the truth, and the life" to the Father, and that "no one comes to the Father" but by him (John 14:6). When they read the Gospel accounts of Jesus' life, they discover that he was both a teacher and a renowned healer and that he passed on this double mission to his apostles, sending them out "to preach the kingdom of God and to heal" (Luke 9:1–2). This mission to preach and to heal is one of the foundations of Catholic health care ministry.

One evening, the evangelist Mark recounts, Jesus was eating in the house of Simon the leper when a woman came to the table and poured a flask of "very costly" nard over his head, anointing him with it. Some of those sitting with him around the table murmured indignantly that "this ointment might have been sold for more than three hundred denarii and given to the poor" (Mark 14:5). It might appear to us a legitimate comment, but it did not so appear to Jesus. He reprimanded them for their thinking: "She has done a beautiful thing to me," he said. "For you always have the poor with you and, whenever you will, you can do good to them; but you will not always have me" (Mark 14:6–7). We ask what Jesus' comment that we will always have the poor with us has to do with Catholic health care, and we answer that it has everything to do with it. The poor, "the uninsured and the underinsured, children and the unborn, single parents, the elderly, those with incurable diseases and chemical dependencies, racial minorities, immigrants and refugees" (*ERD*, 9), the unemployed and underpaid, the homeless—all have a claim on Catholic health care, and that claim is divinely mandated.

Poverty is not a new reality in human experience, and neither is the scandalous inequality between rich and poor. We would expect it, therefore, to feature in the ancient scriptural sources of Catholic ethics, and so it does. To understand the meanings of the ideas expressed in those scriptures, we must first understand the differences between the culture of their times and the culture of our times. American culture today tends to be individualistic, holding to the impossible ideal that individuals should be able to stand unaided on their own two feet. The Mediterranean culture in which the scriptures were written was and is quite different. It values not individualism but community, belonging to some family, some tribe, some society, and the members of a family, a tribe, or a society are honor bound to help the other members, including economically. Two principles, one anthropological, the other theological, underlie everything both the Old and New Testaments say about poverty and wealth. The anthropological principle is a principle of belonging to a tribe or society, most fundamentally to a nuclear family in which parents and their children are bound tightly together as mother, father, brothers, and sisters. The theological principle is that everything in the world that the God of Israel created belongs to God, and women and men are only stewards of what they own.

In ancient Israel that fundamental family belonging was extended to embrace as brothers and sisters all members of Israelite society, and the followers of Jesus (initially all Israelites, remember) extended family kinship to embrace all those who believed in Jesus as the Christ, the anointed one of God, and embraced each other as brothers and sisters (Matt. 25:40; Luke 6:41–42; 1 Cor. 8:13). This pattern is very much in evidence in both the Old and New Testaments' comments about poverty and the obligation of Jews and Christians to care for the poor. They are both called to respond to God's saving actions in human experience with ethical actions in their own experience, specified by the observance of God's commandments. When we ask what those actions are to be, both the Jewish and Christian scriptures leave us in no doubt. The Old Testament reveals that the power of the God who led Israel from slavery in Egypt continues in defense of contemporary "slaves," the defenseless and vulnerable poor. God is "father of the fatherless and protector of widows. . . . God gives the desolate a home to dwell in" (Ps. 68:5–6). To know God is not, as it is in ancient Greece and modern America, to know *that* God is and *what* God is; it is to act like God. To know God as Father of the poor is to act on behalf of the poor. Deuteronomy instructs,

> You shall remember that you were a slave in Egypt and the Lord your God redeemed you from there; therefore, I command you to do this. When you reap your harvest in your field and have forgotten a sheaf in the field, you shall not go back to get it; it shall be for the sojourner, the fatherless, the widow; that the Lord your God may bless you in all the works of your hands. When you beat your olive trees, you shall not go over the boughs again; it shall be for the sojourner, the fatherless, the widow. (Deut. 24:18–22)

In short, take care of the poor.

What Jewish Jesus in the New Testament would later advance as a reciprocal relationship between God and "the least of these my brothers" (Matt. 25:40) has always been embedded in his Jewish tradition as a reciprocal relationship between God and the poor and vulnerable. The prophets consistently link these two and proclaim that to truly know and love God demands action on behalf of the poor and against every injustice perpetrated against them. Jeremiah proclaims this prophetic message: "Thus, says the Lord of Hosts, the God of Israel. Amend your ways and your doings. . . . For if you truly amend your ways and your doings, if you truly execute justice one with another, if you do not oppress the alien, the fatherless, the widow [in other words, the poor] . . . then I will let you dwell in this place, in the land that I gave of old to your fathers forever" (Jer. 7:2–7). The reciprocation could not be made clearer: knowledge and love of God is proved in practice by action on behalf of justice for the poor, vulnerable, and excluded. The book of Proverbs offers an axiomatic statement about this preferential option for the poor: "He who mocks the poor insults his Creator" (Prov. 17:5).

The confession of the followers of Jesus was and is that he is the promised Messiah, in Greek the Christ (Mark 1:1; Matt. 1:1), the one anointed by God "to bring good tidings to the afflicted." Like every good Jew of his time Jesus upheld the reciprocal relationship between God and the poor and insisted that to know and love God is to love and act on behalf of the poor, and to act against every injustice perpetrated against them. Matthew makes this position clear in his Sermon on the Mount: "Not everyone who *says* to me 'Lord, Lord' shall enter the kingdom of heaven but the one who *does* the will of my Father who is in heaven" (Matt. 7:21). That will is to care for the poor. The disciples who responded to Jesus' invitation to "follow me" (Mark 1:17; Matt. 4:19), and that includes every person today who claims to be a Catholic, including every Catholic health care professional, are necessarily committed to the care of the poor. From its very beginning, the *ERD* interprets this biblical mandate correctly. "The biblical mandate to care for the poor," it decrees, "requires us to express this in concrete actions at all levels of Catholic health care" (*ERD*, dir. 2; see also dir. 3) Matthew makes the penalty for not following this mandate clear in his chilling final judgment scene:

> Then he will say to those at his left hand "depart from me you cursed into the eternal fire prepared for the devil and his angels; for I was hungry and you gave me no food, I was thirsty and you gave me no drink, I was a stranger and you did not welcome me, sick and in prison and you did not visit me." Then they will answer, "Lord, when did we see you hungry or thirsty or a stranger or naked or sick or in prison and did not minister to you?" Then he will answer them, "Truly I say to you, as you did it not to one of the least of these, you did it not to me." (Matt. 25:41–45)

The seriousness of the biblical mandate to care for the poor and excluded could not be made clearer. But to make it clearer the Second Vatican Council decreed, "Feed the man dying of hunger, because if you have not fed him you have killed him" (*GS*, 13). That is easily translated into "cure the man dying of cancer," or of drug addiction, or of any other sickness. The Catholic Church has never doubted that faith is proved in actions, and that is what Catholic health care is all about.

The New Testament highlights another Christian behavior intimately related to the reciprocation between God and God's poor. That behavior is one of service to others, especially to the poor and excluded, which Jesus exemplifies in his life and unceasingly strives to inculcate in his disciples. The Gospel Christ articulates this perspective unequivocally: "The Son of Man came not to be served but to serve and to give his life as a ransom for many" (Mark 10:45; Matt. 20:28). Service of others is Christ's way, truth, and life (John 14:6), and service of others is what he strives to inculcate in his disciples of every generation. He instructs them that "whoever would be great among you must be your servant, and whoever would be first among you must be the slave of all" (Mark 10:42–44; Matt. 20:25–27), and he showed them how to be servant by washing his disciples', feet at his Last Supper with them (John 13:5–9). Catholic health care is an obvious manifestation of that Christian service.

The fundamental purpose of productivity, *Gaudium et Spes* advises, "must not be profit or domination. Rather it must be the *service* of man [and woman] and, indeed, of the whole man . . . and every group of men of whatever race and from whatever part of the world" (*GS*, 64). It continues: "If the demands of justice and equity are to be satisfied, vigorous efforts must be made . . . to remove as quickly as possible the immense inequalities which now exist" (*GS*, 66). Those immense inequalities are starkly highlighted by the fact that "while an enormous mass of people still lack the absolute necessities of life, some, even in less advanced countries, live sumptuously or squander wealth. Luxury and misery rub shoulders" (*GS*, 63). Present-day Catholics must shoulder a share of blame for this situation. There are even some, comfortably rich, who chastise Pope Francis for his support of the poor and who invite him to return to the business of the Gospel. They must never have read the clear Gospel teaching we have just exposed or else they have chosen to ignore it.

The commitment of Catholics to the service of the poor has continued to the present day, not only in health care but also in social care for the uninsured and the underinsured, children and the unborn, single parents, the elderly, those with incurable diseases and chemical dependencies, racial minorities, immigrants and refugees, the unemployed and underpaid, the homeless, and all the other excluded in our society. The theologians who have most detailed this Catholic commitment and its connection to Church communion, eucharistic communion, and everyday life are the liberation theologians of South America. These theologians correctly interpret the biblical mandate we have highlighted as a preferential option for the poor, an option that was embraced as a Catholic Church doctrine at two synods of the South American Catholic Church, at

Medellín, Colombia (1968), and Puebla, Mexico (1979). It is no surprise that Pope Francis, a South American, would highlight this doctrine in his papal words and actions. Among the signs of authentic Catholicity, South American bishops taught, is "preferential love and concern for the poor." They pledged themselves and their Churches to make clear through their lives and values and actions that their preference is to serve the poor. Francis speaks out of a dominant biblical tradition and the best of the Catholic tradition when he teaches that "alleviating the grave evil of poverty must be at the very heart of the Church's mission. It is neither optional nor secondary."[21] The questions being asked today about his "novel" words and actions with respect to a Church of the poor and a poor Church are all already answered for those who have paid close attention to the gospels.

Pope John Paul II draws attention to a temptation that Catholics "have not always known how to avoid," the temptation to separate their Catholic faith from their everyday life, to separate their acceptance of the Gospel from "the actual living of the gospel in various situations in the world."[22] The pope implies that, to be faithful to their vocation to follow Jesus the Christ, Catholics need to reach out in active love to the people around them, preferentially as always to the poor and excluded. That demand originates not in the teaching of Pope John Paul II or Pope Francis but in the teaching of Jesus the Christ and the Catholic tradition that follows him as servant of God's poor and excluded. John Paul and Francis do no more than authentically interpret the ancient Jewish-Christian scriptural mandate for the situations of their times and places. Francis writes, "How can it be that it is not a news item when an elderly homeless person dies of exposure, but it is news when the stock market loses two points? This is a case of exclusion. Can we continue to stand by when food is thrown away while people are starving? This is a case of inequality" (EG, 53). *Gaudium et Spes* has the final word here:

> Mindful of the Lord's saying: "By this will all men know that you are my disciples, if you have love for one another" (John 13:35), Catholics cannot yearn for anything more ardently than to serve the men [and women] of the modern world ever more generously and effectively. . . . Not everyone who cries "Lord, Lord" will enter into the kingdom of heaven, but those who do the Father's will and take a strong grip on the job at hand. (GS, 93)

The job at hand for contemporary Catholics, perhaps especially for Catholic health care professionals, is the job of once again anointing the risen Jesus, this time not with expensive nard or empty political words but with the actions of a faith that sees injustice and does justice for God's poor and excluded, in imitation of the Christ they profess to follow.

SUGGESTED READING

International Theological Commission. "Theology Today: Perspectives, Principles and Criteria." Roma: Libreria Editrice Vaticana, 2011.

McElroy, Robert W. "A Church for the Poor." *America*, October 21, 2013.

McIntosh, Mark A. *Discernment and Truth: The Spirituality and Theology of Knowledge*. New York: Herder and Herder, 2004.

Salzman, Todd A., and Michael G. Lawler. *Introduction to Catholic Theological Ethics: Foundations and Applications*. Maryknoll, NY: Orbis, 2019.

Schneiders, Sandra M. "Religion and Spirituality: Strangers, Rivals, or Partners?" The Santa Clara Lectures 6 (2000).

Tracey, David. *Gods and Diseases: Making Sense of Our Physical and Mental Wellbeing*. London: Routledge, 2011.

NOTES

1. Sandra M. Schneiders, "Religion and Spirituality: Strangers, Rivals, or Partners?" The Santa Clara Lectures 6 (2000), 1.

2. Schneiders, 4–5.

3. David Tracey, *Gods and Diseases: Making Sense of Our Physical and Mental Wellbeing* (London: Routledge, 2011), 194, 195.

4. See DeCosse and Nairn, *Conscience and Catholic Health Care*.

5. Thomas Aquinas, IV Sent., dist. 38, art. 4.

6. Joseph Ratzinger, "Introductory Article and Chapter 1: The Dignity of the Human Person," in *Commentary on the Documents of Vatican II*, vol. 5, ed. Herbert Vorgrimler (New York: Herder, 1969), 115–63, at 134.

7. Cardinal Newman, "Letter to the Duke of Norfolk," 1875, available at http://www.newmanreader.org/works/anglicans/volume2/gladstone/section5.html.

8. International Theological Commission, "Sensus Fidei in the Life of the Church," 2, 4.

9. International Theological Commission, "Theology Today."

10. Lonergan, *Method in Theology*, 217.

11. Pascal Wallisch, "Two Years Later, We Finally Know Why People Saw 'The Dress' Differently," *Slate*, April 12, 2017, available at https://slate.com/technology/2017/04/heres-why-people-saw-the-dress-differently.html.

12. Lonergan, *Insight*, 344. See also Lonergan, *Method in Theology*, 217–19.

13. Mark A. McIntosh, *Discernment and Truth: The Spirituality and Theology of Knowledge* (New York: Herder and Herder, 2004), 8.

14. Jeffrey M. Schwartz and Sharon Begley, *The Mind and the Brain: Neuroplasticity and the Power of Mental Force* (New York: Harper, 2002), 294.

15. Schwartz and Begley, 295.

16. Schwartz and Begley, 324–25.

17. Schwartz and Begley, 360.

18. Selling, "*Gaudium et Spes*," 151.

19. Brown, "Experience and Development," 300.

20. Lisa Sowle Cahill, *Sex, Gender, and Christian Ethics* (Cambridge: Cambridge University Press, 1996), 55.

21. See Bishop Robert W. McElroy, "A Church for the Poor," *America*, October 21, 2013, 13, available at https://www.americamagazine.org/church-poor.

22. John Paul II, *Christifideles Laici*, 2.

CHAPTER SIX

Collaboration between Catholic and Non-Catholic Health Care Institutions

Two fundamental developments in the Catholic Church impact our perspective on the interpretation and application of principles governing cooperation (PGC), one negative and one positive. The negative development is the Catholic sex-abuse crisis and its ecclesiological implications, especially how the crisis impacts the authority of the bishops. The positive development is Pope Francis's Catholic holistic human dignity and new pastoral methods, which include synodality, discernment, and accompaniment.

The revisions in the 2018 *ERD* focus on part 6, "Collaborative Arrangements with Other Health Care Organizations and Providers." One major event that contributed to these revisions was the reconfiguration of Catholic Health West into Dignity Health. Catholic Health West was founded by the Sisters of Mercy in 1986 as a Catholic health care institution that owned and operated Catholic and community hospitals. Its first acquisition of a non-Catholic health care institution was in 1992. In 2012 it became Dignity Health, a non-Catholic health care institution owning and operating both Catholic and community hospitals. It dropped its formal connection to the Roman Catholic Church and changed its name to Dignity Health in part because of a competitive market and concerns that its Catholic affiliation would limit health care delivery services and prevent mergers with non-Catholic health care institutions. Dignity Health carries out direct sterilizations in its health care facilities, but it does not allow abortions or reproductive technologies prohibited in the *ERD*.[1] Given their concerns over the reconfiguration of Catholic Health West to Dignity Health, the USCCB submitted a list of questions (*dubia*) to the Congregation for the Doctrine of the Faith seeking guidance on this collaborative relationship. The

CDF replied in February 2014 with a document titled "Some Principles for Collaboration with Non-Catholic Entities in the Provision of Health Care Services."[2] The response extended beyond the bishops' specific questions and laid out general guidelines for collaborative relationships between Catholic and non-Catholic health care institutions in the United States. The four-page response includes a prologue and seventeen principles. Rather than add the CDF response as an appendix to the existing fifth edition of the *ERD*, the USCCB decided to revise the *ERD* in light of the response and issued the sixth edition of the *ERD* in 2018. The revisions to part 6 propose three changes. First, they strengthen the authority of the local bishop and more clearly articulate his role in interpreting and applying the *ERD*, especially on collaborative relationships between Catholic and non-Catholic health care institutions. Second, they provide new directives for such relationships based on the CDF's response. Third, they add a new consideration to PGC and scandal, namely witness, to guide those relationships. In this chapter, we consider and critically analyze each revision.

CRITICAL ANALYSIS OF REVISIONS TO THE *ERD*

Bishops and Authority in the *ERD*

In its commentary on the revised *ERD*, the National Catholic Bioethics Center highlights the *ERD*'s focus on "the authority of the diocesan Bishop," noting that even though a bishop's authority over ministries in his diocese is "well recognized in canon law" and has been consistently noted in the *ERD* since the 1994 edition, "this strong statement is a notable addition in the new edition" and is reflected in the final paragraph of the introduction to part 6 and in directives 67–69.[3] That paragraph states "the ultimate responsibility for interpreting and applying . . . the directives rests with the diocesan Bishop" (*ERD*, 25). This emphasis on the bishop's "ultimate responsibility" is one of the many changes in the introduction to part 6.

Drawing from directive 71 in the fifth edition, directive 67 includes the bishop's responsibility to determine whether collaborative relationships include wrongful cooperation or give scandal or, an added third criterion, "undermine the Church's witness." Directive 68 draws from the fifth edition's directives 67 and 68 and emphasizes both the need to consult with the bishop "in a timely manner" regarding collaborative relationships that may affect the Catholic identity of a health care institution or cause scandal and the bishop's approval for collaborative relationships for institutions within his jurisdiction.

Directive 69 is entirely new. It includes four components from principle 17 of the CDF statement and adds a fifth component: 1) recognition that the bishop must be informed of agreements or cessation of agreements involving Catholic health care institutions within his jurisdiction, 2) recognition of the need for the bishop's authorization of such agreements, 3) recognition that Catholic health care institutions can span multiple dioceses, 4) recognition that the bishop in the diocese where the system's headquarters are located must collaborate with bishops in other dioceses where affiliated institutions are located, and 5) recognition that "the Bishops involved in this collaboration should make every effort to reach a consensus" (*ERD*, dir. 69). Nowhere in directive 69, or anywhere else in the *ERD*, are guidelines offered for reaching this consensus. The introduction to part 6 specifies that when forming such collaborative relationships "Catholic leaders" must, among other criteria, abide by canon law. As we noted in chapter 4, however, canon law is ambiguous on providing guidelines for resolving possible conflicts between bishops and, since neither the USCCB nor the CDF's statement provide specific guidelines, guidelines are left ambiguous and at the discretion of individual bishops who exercise "ultimate responsibility" for all decisions with respect to the *ERD*.

Bishops and Authority in the *ERD*: A Critique

One may reasonably ask, if the bishop's authority is emphasized in tradition, codified in canon law, and recognized in earlier editions of the *ERD*, why make this authority such a focus in the revised *ERD*? There are several plausible responses to this question. First, health care delivery systems are becoming more competitive and complex. They involve Catholic and non-Catholic health care institutions and government programs and regulations, such as those reflected in the Affordable Care Act, that provide or mandate services contrary to the *ERD*, including contraceptives, abortifacients, and direct sterilizations. This situation may be seen within the USCCB as a threat to Catholic health care institutions' identity and mission. Emphasizing the bishops' authority for determining collaborative relationships is an attempt to respond to this threat.

Second, many bishops see the move toward secularism as a direct threat to religious liberty and feel the need to respond with strong statements on, and institutional identity that protects, religious liberty. One way of doing this is to reassert the authority of the bishops and their duty to protect religious liberty and individual consciences in health care decisions. However, we suggest, this is a specious argument. Research data on where Catholics stand on Catholic teachings the bishops defend, such as teachings absolutely prohibiting contraception, direct sterilization, artificial reproductive technologies, and abortion, reveal that the consciences of the majority of Catholics are not in line with official Catholic teaching. By mandating prohibitions against certain procedures that many Catholics and other people of good will disagree with in good conscience, the bishops are actually violating those consciences and religious liberty. The question arises then, *whose* religious liberty is being defended, and what is the relationship between individual consciences and institutional identity? Third, as discussed in chapter 1, at the root of the Phoenix case seems to be Bishop Olmsted's emphasis on episcopal authority and the fact that Saint Joseph's leadership did not conform to his authority on an abortion case, regardless of the medical, ethical, legal, and theological arguments presented to defend Saint Joseph's action. Fourth, and perhaps most significant, the USCCB's need to emphasize the bishops' authority in the *ERD* could be linked to the bishops' loss of authority and moral credibility due to the Catholic sex-abuse scandal and their handling of it.[4] It is to that consideration and its implications for the Church in general and the *ERD* in specific that we turn.

Sex Abuse, Authority, and an Ecclesial Paradigm Shift

The paradigm of the CDF's statement and the *ERD* is a hierarchical ecclesiology that continues to promote the bishop's authority with or without consultation of divergent voices. Anyone who doubts that ecclesiology is spiritually dangerous doctrine need only consider the Crusades, Inquisition, institutional corruption throughout history, and the present sex-abuse crisis and its cover-up by bishops. This latter event, we suggest, cries out for conversion and an ecclesiological paradigm shift. As the CDF notes in its statement on principles for collaboration between Catholic and non-Catholic health care institutions, "It is precisely the decisions of individuals that determine the identity and moral character of an institution."[5] This statement needs to be applied not only to Catholic health care institutions and their administrators but also to the institutional Church itself. The decision of many bishops, like Cardinal Theodore McCarrick, to commit and/or cover up sexual abuse has fundamentally damaged their individual and collective authority and that of the Church itself. Neil Ormerod correctly notes that the abuse crisis has caused "a crisis of episcopal authority as lay Catholics [and society at large] have lost trust in the office of the Bishop."[6] Importantly, it is a loss of trust not only in *individual* bishops who committed or covered up sexual abuse but also in the bishops' *office* itself and in its ability to exercise credible authority on religious and moral matters. The loss of trust and credibility profoundly impacts the bishops' authority and the faithful's and general public's perception of individual bishops and of the USCCB when they seek to assert their authority, including on collaborative relationships between Catholic and non-Catholic health care institutions. To understand this crisis of authority and authenticity Ormerod, drawing from Bernard Lonergan and Joseph Komonchak, explores the social nature of authority.[7]

Lonergan adopts Max Weber's concept of "legitimate authority," expanding that concept to include a normative dimension grounded in human authenticity. For Lonergan, the source of power in legitimate authority derives from the cooperation between communities that share values and meanings; authenticity "confers on power the aura and prestige of authority. Unauthenticity leaves power naked. It reveals power as mere power. Similarly, authenticity legitimates authorities, and unauthenticity destroys their authority and reveals them as merely powerful."[8] Lonergan makes a further distinction between authority and authorities. Although authority is shared with the entire community, authorities are those who have been entrusted with particular offices and delegated with particular powers. External criteria, deduced from a community's shared meanings and values, legitimate and guide authorities. These criteria, though necessary, are not sufficient. To be sufficient, they must include authenticity as well. Moral authenticity requires God's grace and is grounded in personal holiness.[9] In the ongoing sex-abuse crisis, many bishops violated communal meanings, values, and personal holiness, all of which fundamentally damaged their authority and authenticity individually and collectively.

Komonchak embraces Weber's definition of authority and applies it to teaching authority. Legitimate teaching authority is "trustworthy power."[10] The trustworthiness of power associated with an office is contingent on the trustworthiness of the people holding that office. For Lonergan, the authenticity of the office is dependent on the authenticity of the office holders. When the office holders violate trust, as many bishops did in the cover-up of the sex-abuse scandal, the office itself loses its trustworthiness and, therefore, its authenticity as a trustworthy power. This is where individual bishops' violation of trust has led the Church. The lack of authenticity in individual bishops who covered up the sex-abuse scandal has resulted in a lack of authenticity in the episcopal office in general. This lack of authenticity in individual bishops and in the episcopal offices they occupy, and its impact on the faithful, applies not only to how they have addressed the sex-abuse crisis but extends also to the entire Church and its ecclesial ministries, including the authority of individual bishops to determine collaborative relationships in health care. The lack of authority, authenticity, trust, and credibility invite a fundamental ecclesial paradigm shift to restore authority and authenticity and to rebuild trust and credibility.

As a body, the USCCB appears to be unaware that the sex-abuse crisis, and the organization's handling of it, has reduced its own authenticity and legitimacy as an authority. It seems to believe that it can isolate this violation of power and trust, grounded in a hierarchical ecclesiology, and continue with

business as usual in all other areas of authority. Authority, however, cannot isolate its misdeeds to one area and act as if no other area is affected. Authenticity
is not an isolated reality. Any violation of authenticity permeates the whole
perception of authority and how that authority is carried out in every area, not
just in the area where authenticity was violated. When it comes to collaboration between Catholic and non-Catholic health care institutions, "the ultimate
responsibility for interpreting and applying . . . the directives rests with the diocesan Bishop" (*ERD*, 25). Given the sex-abuse crisis and the damage it has done
to bishops' authenticity as moral leaders within the Church, and in light of the
anthropological and methodological contributions Pope Francis has made on
how the Church can do theological ethics, it is perplexing and even scandalous
that the USCCB would not take these insights into consideration when revising
the *ERD* and incorporate them into those revisions. This lack of insight reflects
serious episcopal *scotosis* about the fundamental ecclesial impact of the sex-abuse
crisis and also calls for an ecclesial paradigm shift.

Synodality, Discernment, and Accompaniment

Pope Francis's emphasis on synodality and its related concepts, discernment
and accompaniment, could facilitate the ecclesial paradigm shift we call for
and serve to restore the bishop's moral authority and credibility.[11] We discussed
synodality in some detail in chapter 4, and here we underscore some of its aspects to highlight our call for synodality to guide how we understand episcopal
authority in a communional rather than a hierarchical ecclesiology and how
such a shift impacts the discernment of collaborative relationships between
Catholic and non-Catholic health care institutions. Pope Francis emphasizes
the *sensus fidelium* as an essential dimension of synodality: "The presence of the
Spirit gives Christians a certain connaturality with divine realities, and a wisdom which enables them to grasp those realities intuitively, even when they lack
the wherewithal to give them precise expression" (*EG*, 119). Drawing from Francis, the International Theological Commission emphasizes the need for synodality in the Church: "The emergence of a new climate in . . . a more careful
discernment of the advanced demands of modern consciousness concerning
the participation of every citizen in running society call for a new and deeper
experience and presentation of the mystery of the Church as intrinsically synodal."[12] The notion of a communion Church, the *sensus fidelium*, and Catholic
social teaching's principle of subsidiarity all emphasize the inclusion of all the
faithful in every process of dialogue in the Church.

The communion, synodal church extends back to the earliest foundations of
the Church and was articulated by Cyprian of Carthage in the third century:
"While nothing should be done in the local Church without the bishop, it is

equally true that nothing should be done without your council (the Presbyters & Deacons)—or without the consensus of the people, always holding firm to the rule according to which the episcopate is one, of which each member has an undivided share in it."[13] Up until the twelfth century, this earliest model of Church included the faithful in the selection of bishops.[14] The participation of the laity in this way is a necessary corrective from a hierarchical-clerical Church to a communional-synodal Church that would help bishops retrieve authority and authenticity. The ITC summarizes this historical synodal model thus: "The dynamic of synodality thus joins the communitarian aspect which includes the whole People of God, the collegial dimension that is part of the exercise of episcopal ministry, and the primatial ministry of the Bishop of Rome."[15] To have an undivided share in the episcopate, there must be structures in place to ensure that the voices of all people of good will can be heard, including professionals in Catholic hospitals that serve diverse religious, racial, and cultural populations.

According to the *ERD*, collaborative relationships must be determined according to Church teaching, natural law, and canon law (*ERD*, 23). The participation of people of good will in discerning the content of natural law through the process of synodality would affect discernment of what is morally acceptable and unacceptable in collaborative relationships. The principle of synodality in discernment requires dialogue with people who agree *and* disagree with a particular perspective, even with the perspective of a bishop who is presenting church teaching on a specific ethical issue. Pope Francis wisely summarizes this process: "Keep an open mind. Don't get bogged down in your own limited ideas and opinions but be prepared to change or expand them. The combination of two different ways of thinking can lead to a synthesis that enriches both" (*AL*, 139). Consulting only with "approved authors" risks reinforcing the status quo without due discussion. Francis's proposal reflects synodal dialogue and a fundamental paradigm shift from a hierarchical-clerical to a communion-synodal model of Church.

Accompaniment emphasizes not an absolute adherence to natural law norms but journeying with the other in the physical, psychological, emotional, spiritual, and relational dimensions of Catholic holistic human development. It resists absolute norms that limit the witness of Christ's care, compassion, and mercy that is foundational to Catholic health care. Pope Francis wisely notes a principle of Saint Thomas Aquinas, cited for the first time in a papal pronouncement:

Although there is necessity in the general principles [Christ's healing ministry], the more we descend to matters of detail [in particular health care situations, for instance] the more frequently we encounter defects. . . . In matters of action, truth or practical rectitude is not the same for all, as to matters of detail, but only as to the general principles; and where there is the same rectitude in matters of detail, it is not equally known to all. . . . The principle will be found to fail, according as we descend further into detail. (*AL*, 304; *ST*, I–II, q. 94, art. 4)

The details of people's health care decisions require discernment and accompaniment, not a blind application of norms that may or may not be relevant to the values or meanings of a particular patient. When it comes to absolute norms, discernment and accompaniment require inductive reasoning, interpretation, and application, not an absolute, deductive institutional mandate.

The paradigm shift to a synodal-communion Church presents a foundational critique of the current *ERD* and its emphasis on the bishop's authority and has profound implications for future revisions of the *ERD*. First, it redefines the bishop's authority from a focus on his "ultimate responsibility" to a focus on "servant leadership" that promotes collaboration through synodality, discernment, and accompaniment. Servant leadership begins with synodality, discernment, and accompaniment to reach responsible decision-making on collaborative relationships. It does not begin with an assertion of bishops' authority that dispenses with the process of synodality. Second, it provides principled guidelines for bishops to "reach a consensus" when discerning collaborative relationships of health care systems that span multiple dioceses. The ITC summarizes these guidelines as "the integration of the exercise of collegiality by and the synodality lived by the whole People of God as an expression of communion between local Churches within the universal Church."[16] This integration will require a deliberate and sustained effort to both create Church structures that promote synodality among all the people of God and work toward building trust to establish authentic leadership in the Church. This paradigmatic shift from a hierarchical-clerical to a communional-synodal approach to decision-making in the Church will have implications for the interpretation and application of PGC.

The Principles Governing Cooperation

The inclusion of an explanation of PGC is a fundamental revision of the *ERD*. The principles were explained in the appendix to the 1994 edition, but that explanation was not included in the 2001 and 2009 editions due, in part, to concerns about their inaccurate interpretation and application that allowed cooperation with non-Catholic health care institutions that performed procedures deemed to be immoral. PGC are perhaps the most difficult principles in the Catholic moral tradition to apply to concrete situations.[17] They were formulated traditionally in the manuals of moral theology and applied to individuals and their actions to determine if participating in the action of another was morally justified. The *ERD* extends them to institutions, and they assist us in judging whether the complex collaborative relationships between Catholic and non-Catholic health care institutions are morally right or wrong. In this section, we present the *ERD*'s understanding of PGC and its condemnation of "intrinsically immoral [actions such as] abortion, euthanasia, assisted suicide, and direct sterilization" in directive 70, then consider terms, concepts, and perspectives that impact their interpretation and application in collaborative relationships.

The *ERD* explains PGC, distinguished as formal and material cooperation, to determine whether collaboration between Catholic and non-Catholic health care institutions can be justified. Formal cooperation in wrongdoing "occurs when an action, either by its very nature or by the form it takes in a concrete situation, can be defined as a direct participation in an [immoral] act . . . or a sharing in the immoral intention of the person committing it." Formal cooperation exists either when the wrongdoer and the cooperator share the same intention or "when the cooperator directly participates in the immoral act, even if the cooperator does not share the intention of the wrongdoer, but participates as a means to some other end." Formal cooperation can include "authorizing wrongdoing, approving it, prescribing it, actively defending it, or giving specific direction about carrying it out" (*ERD*, 24). If the cooperation is formal, it is always immoral.

Material cooperation focuses on the object of the act and occurs when the cooperator "contributes to the immoral activity in a way that is causally related but not essential to the immoral act itself" (*ERD*, 24). The *ERD* distinguishes between immediate and mediate material cooperation. The appendix to the 1994 edition explained the distinction between the two, but the revised 2018 edition offers no explanation. Immediate material cooperation is "when the object of the cooperator is the same as the object of the wrongdoer" (*ERD* [1994], appendix). It is morally the same as implicit formal cooperation unless there is duress. The 1994 *ERD* included a discussion of duress to distinguish between immediate material cooperation that could be justified and implicit formal cooperation that could not be justified. Mediate material cooperation, which can be moral, occurs "when the object of the cooperator's action remains distinguishable from that of the wrongdoer's" (*ERD* [1994], appendix). The explanatory appendix was left out of the 2001 and 2009 editions, and the 2001 edition explained the omission: "Experience has shown that the brief articulation of the principles of cooperation that was presented [in the 1994 edition] . . . did not sufficiently forestall certain possible misinterpretations and in practice gave rise to problems in concrete applications of the principles." Kelly notes, however, a more specific rationale for the omission that the bishops do not include. The 1994 *ERD* allowed immediate material cooperation in cases of duress; the 2001, 2009, and 2018 editions forbid immediate material cooperation with acts that are intrinsically immoral (dir. 70). The later editions remove the circumstance of duress that justifies immediate material cooperation between Catholic and non-Catholic health care institutions in intrinsically evil acts such as direct sterilizations. The 1994 edition and subsequent editions are in sharp contrast and at odds with one another on whether, and in what circumstances, immediate material cooperation can be justified.[18]

The 2018 *ERD* offers a brief explanation of PGC but does not include a discussion of proximate and remote material cooperation, though it mentions that the causal relationship between the act of the wrongdoer and cooperator must be evaluated. "Duress" (*ERD* [1994], appendix) and "grave pressure" (CDF, Principles) that might justify material cooperation are not specifically discussed. Instead, the revised *ERD* broadens the criteria to justify material cooperation, including "whether the cooperator's act is morally good or neutral in itself, how significant is its causal contribution to the wrongdoer's act, how serious is the immoral act of the wrongdoer, and how important are the goods to be preserved or the harms to be avoided by cooperating" (*ERD*, 24). We add to that list the discernment of the hierarchy of both goods and harms in a particular situation of cooperation.

The National Catholic Bioethics Center notes that directive 70 is the only directive in Part Six that was not revised from the fifth edition. In this directive, the *ERD* focuses on intrinsically evil acts—abortion, euthanasia, assisted suicide, and direct sterilization—and asserts that Catholic health care institutions cannot engage in immediate material cooperation with non-Catholic institutions that perform such acts. The Bioethics Center maintains that this directive, supported as it is by authoritative magisterial teachings in the footnotes, must be "a high priority in assessing any collaborative relationship."[19] The emphasis on intrinsically evil acts as the most important consideration for discerning collaborative relationships distinguishes different perspectives on the interpretation and application of PGC.

Considerations in Interpreting and Applying the *ERD*

Before exploring PGC and how they may guide collaborative relationships between Catholic and non-Catholic health care institutions, we must first explore some tensions between the origins of the principles and their current application.

PENANCE, INDIVIDUALS, AND THE PRINCIPLES GOVERNING COOPERATION

Catholic moral theology originated as a science for administering the sacrament of penance. Its focus, especially since the Council of Trent and the formation of the seminary system, was to train priests to administer the sacrament of penance. That training was focused on the penitents' acts, their number, severity, and circumstances, with a view to determining the nature and gravity of their sins and a just penance and forgiveness. This created an individualistic, act-focused, sin-centered moral theology that permeated Catholic thinking on moral theology in general, including PGC.

An important issue addressed in the manuals was whether it was morally acceptable for a cooperator to knowingly or intentionally cooperate in the wrongful act of another person, the primary moral agent. Degrees of cooperation were recognized and, depending on the knowledge, intentionality, and causality of that cooperation, the cooperator could be more or less morally culpable. For instance, a physician who refers a woman to an abortion clinic for an abortion may have a high degree of sinful cooperation in the abortion, but a nurse who cares for a woman who has had an abortion may have a negligible or no degree of sinful cooperation in the abortion. The role of the confessor was to discern the nature and severity—formal or material, immediate or mediate, and proximate or remote—of cooperation and moral culpability in order to administer the sacrament in a just and loving manner.

In its response to the USCCB's *dubia*, the CDF notes that cooperation "is ultimately about actions of individual human beings" (principle 1). Rather than focusing on individual persons cooperating with other individual persons in wrongdoing, however, the *ERD* focuses on institutions cooperating with other institutions in wrongdoing. It does not clearly distinguish between individuals and institutions, but it does note that collaborative relationships, among other considerations, should "abide by canon law" (*ERD*, 25), which distinguishes between physical, moral, and juridic persons. A physical person is an individual person created in the image of God and endowed with human dignity, the very foundation of Catholic ethical teaching. A moral person is "a group or succession of natural persons who are united by a common purpose and, hence, who have a particular relationship to each other and who, because of that relationship, may be conceived of as a single entity" and, therefore, as a moral agent.[20] A juridic person is a moral person with recognized status in the Church with corresponding canonical obligations and rights according to its nature.[21] A Catholic health care institution may be both a moral and a juridic person subject to canonical obligations and rights.[22]

The *ERD* notes that "assessing material cooperation can be complex, and legitimate disagreements may arise over which factors are most relevant in a given case" (*ERD*, 24). Important questions for PGC to determine are whether material cooperation between Catholic and non-Catholic health care institutions is morally acceptable and whether the distinction between a physical and a juridic person has moral implications for interpreting and applying the principles. We note several distinctions between individuals and institutions that may affect their interpretation and application in cases of immediate material cooperation. First, individuals and institutions may both engage in material participation over an extended period, but in cases where the justification for material cooperation is no longer present, it is more difficult for an institution than for an individual to withdraw from that cooperative arrangement. This may create a higher ethical bar for institutional than individual material cooperation. Second, the concern with scandal, a criterion we discuss in detail later in this chapter, may be greater for institutions than for individuals. One of the criteria the *ERD* includes for determining material cooperation is a consideration of the benefits and harms of a collaborative, contractual relationship. Cathleen Kaveny comments that the shift from applying PGC from individuals to institutions transfers the focus from the harm to be avoided in the case of an individual to the benefit to be achieved in the case of an institution.[23]

A fundamental benefit of health care institutions is extending health care and Christ's healing ministry as far as possible while minimizing any possible harm. It seems to us that scandal, which is a consideration for measuring harm, can be easily addressed by explaining the benefits gained from immediate material cooperation with non-Catholic institutions that carry out procedures deemed immoral. The explanation can emphasize the positive moral obligation to extend health care to as many people as possible while still reiterating Catholic teaching against procedures deemed immoral. In other words, the benefits of providing health care and promoting Jesus' healing ministry in a non-Catholic health care institution might alleviate moral concerns about the violation of one of the Church's absolute norms.

An additional consideration in the historical development of PGC is the context for interpreting and applying them. The manuals, which interpreted and applied the principles, focused on individuals who were Catholic and lived in a cultural context in which it was widely accepted that, for instance, abortion, sterilization, and fornication were immoral.[24] Catholic and non-Catholic health care institutions today are not limited to serving Catholic populations; they serve diverse religious, racial, cultural populations. In addition, many of the Catholics they serve dissent from the Church's teachings on biomedical and sexual ethical issues, and the mores in society reflect a more pluralist and diverse context. These factors combined make it much more difficult to determine what constitutes wrongdoing and what cooperation in wrongdoing looks like.

Such complexity and the reality of pluralism in Catholicism, society, and the complex institutional relationships in health care delivery may need to shift the focus in applying PGC from avoiding cooperation in wrongdoing to promoting cooperation for the realization of the common good.

INDIVIDUAL AND INSTITUTIONAL CONSCIENCE

A second consideration is the role and function of conscience in discerning the interpretation and application of PGC. That role and function is unclear canonically and ethically in a moral and juridic institutional perspective compared to a physical person perspective. Even though the CDF emphasizes that cooperation pertains to individual acts and, therefore, would depend on the individual conscience to discern cooperation, the *ERD* considers what we would call an "institutional conscience,"[25] whereby "Catholic health care does not offend the rights of individual conscience by refusing to provide or permit medical procedures that are judged morally wrong by the teaching authority of the Church" (*ERD*, 8). In the *ERD*, the teaching of the Catholic Church supersedes individual conscience. This raises an important question: in the relationship between individual conscience, institutions, and Church teaching, which takes priority?

In our discussion of anthropology and Catholic holistic human dignity, we demonstrated Pope Francis's return to traditional Catholic teaching on the authority and inviolability of conscience that the *ERD* does not seem to reflect. The *ERD*, like Archbishop Chaput, proposes Church teaching as the objective norm and reduces conscience to the subjective realm that must obey that teaching to be a well-informed conscience. In his claim that direct sterilization can never be justified by immediate cooperation in collaborative relationships because it is an intrinsically evil act, Lawrence Welch cites Pope John Paul II's *Veritatis Splendor*, which states that Church teaching contains moral truth which "brings to light the truths which [conscience] ought already to possess" (*VS*, 64).[26] This statement makes two assumptions. First, it assumes that the Church's absolute but not infallible norms are true. As we argued in chapters 2 and 3, the anthropological and methodological justification for many of the Church's absolute sexual norms are debatable and, therefore, so are the claims that the conscience should already possess them. Sociological research demonstrates that a majority of Catholics in the United States do not accept the truth of Church teaching on sexual ethical issues like direct sterilization, abortion when the woman's life is in danger, and physician-assisted suicide.

Second, Welch's quote from *Veritatis Splendor* co-opts conscience and dictates what constitutes an informed conscience.[27] Such co-opting conflicts with the history of Catholic teaching on the authority and inviolability of conscience we treated in the previous chapter. That tradition is evident in Aquinas, John Henry Cardinal Newman, theologian Joseph Ratzinger, *Gaudium et Spes, Dignitatis Humane,* and Pope Francis. "We have been called to form consciences," Francis teaches, "not replace them" (*AL*, 37).

Third, on the relationship between non-infallible Church teaching, which covers all moral teaching in the *ERD*, including its absolute norms that prohibit intrinsically immoral acts, and the Christian faithful, canon law calls for "*religiosum obsequium.*" There is a debate about the translation of the Latin *obsequium*. In the Canon Law Society's official English translation of the *Code* in 1983, *religiosum obsequium* is translated as "religious respect" (canons 752, 753).[28] In its 1997 official English translation of the *Code*, it is translated as "religious submission" (cc. 752, 753).[29] There is a wide gulf between submission and respect, and we endorse theologian Francis Sullivan's reading of *obsequium* as more accurate: "To give the required *obsequium religiosum* to the teaching of the ordinary *Magisterium* means to make an honest and sustained effort to overcome any contrary opinion I might have, and to achieve a sincere assent of my mind to this teaching."[30] This translation allows for conscientious and legitimate dissent from non-infallible teaching, which applies to both Catholic social and sexual teaching. Although bishops tolerate dissent from Catholic social teaching, they show no toleration for dissent from Catholic sexual teaching. There are inconsistencies in ecclesial perspectives on different types of church teaching; the anthropology and method underlying that teaching; the authority, role, and function of the teaching in relation to individual and institutional conscience; and assessing cooperation.

Exercising religious respect requires that the faithful must avoid two extremes when it comes to Church teaching. First, they must avoid ecclesiastical positivism and blind obedience to magisterial teaching that assumes bishops have access to knowledge of the natural law that other believers do not have. The long-held teachings on usury, slavery, and religious freedom, now magisterially recognized as false, remind us to take caution here.[31] Second, the faithful must also avoid total disregard for magisterial teaching, given the promise of the Holy Spirit to guide the Church into all truth. There is a presumption of truth in Church teaching, but that presumption does not rule out dissent from teaching on the basis of the authority of a well-formed conscience. Dissent must be possible given the fact that the magisterium has been in error in the past and can be mistaken in the present.[32]

How does such an understanding of the authority and inviolability of the individual conscience function institutionally in relation to PGC? Neither the *ERD* nor canon law address the idea of a moral and juridic institutional conscience. How are the principles to be interpreted and applied when there are disagreements of well-informed consciences among physical persons that make up a moral and juridic person to discern the truth of Church teaching on specific ethical issues that are being debated in the context of collaboration? Although the *ERD* does not address this specific question, it does assert that the local bishop has the final say in determining such matters. This, however, is an argument from authority and reflects a hierarchical ecclesiology and ecclesiastical positivism; it is not an argument grounded in a communion ecclesiology, synodality, discernment, and accompaniment. It allows for the violation of individual consciences based on a moral and juridic institutional conscience or the bishop's authority. In *Amoris Laetitia*, Pope Francis gives priority to the individual conscience over institutional norms in cases of communion for the divorced and remarried without an annulment. If such prioritization of conscience over the Church's teaching applies in the sacramental life of the Church, it seems that it would also apply in collaborative relationships where individual consciences conflict with the institutional conscience.

Following Josef Fuchs, we propose that conscience has two dimensions: an object orientation and a subject orientation.[33] The former is informed by Church teaching and the other sources of ethical knowledge, scripture, tradition, science, and experience. The latter selects, interprets, prioritizes, and integrates these sources of ethical knowledge in light of the particular social, historical, contextual, relational, and biological dimensions of the human person to discern an informed-conscience decision that facilitates human dignity and the common good. This understanding of conscience embraces different perspectives and may lead people to different conclusions on ethical issues, including those addressed by absolute magisterial norms. We believe institutions maintain similar object-subject orientations collectively. The tension between the "institutional conscience" proposed by the *ERD* and the tradition of PGC that applies to individual conscience must, at least, be acknowledged and addressed in any credible revision of the *ERD*.

Common Good and the *ERD*

To a certain extent, the revised *ERD* has provided an essential hermeneutical ethical principle to bridge the divide between the individual and the institutional and to guide the interpretation and application of PGC. Although the revised edition removed a reference in part 6 to Catholic social teaching (*ERD* [2009], 34), it added three references to the common good (*ERD*, 23). It earlier states that the common good "is realized when economic, political, and social conditions ensure protection for the fundamental rights of all individuals and enable all to fulfill their common purpose and reach their common goals" (*ERD*, 8). The introduction of the common good is crucial in that it shifts the focus from individual acts to the complexity of the individual person as a social being who exists within social structures. The notion of the common good demands consideration of this complexity when discerning collaborative relationships.

There are at least two perspectives on the common good that reflect Catholic identity and affect how the principles governing cooperation can be interpreted and applied in collaborative relationships.[34] The first perspective, represented by Cardinal Burke and others, focuses on absolute norms and intrinsically immoral acts to discern whether cooperation is morally acceptable.[35] In his discussion of voting and cooperation, Burke presents a clear hierarchy of values and asserts that the common good must realize and protect what he calls "the economy of life," "the inviolable dignity of human life, the integrity of marital union, and the free exercise of conscience."[36] The *ERD* lists abortion, euthanasia, assisted suicide, and direct sterilization as intrinsically immoral acts that do not permit immediate material cooperation by Catholic health care institutions. Protecting and realizing these values is foundational to the common good and a just society and should be prioritized before any other value.

Regarding possible mergers or partnerships between Catholic and non-Catholic health care institutions, Burke asks, "Why would a Catholic hospital see the need to compete for secular prestige by engaging in practices which violate the moral law? The unique contribution and therefore prestige of a Catholic healthcare institution comes from its fidelity to the Church's teaching in every aspect of its life." This absolutist stance on a strict hierarchy of values seems to rule out the possibility of immediate material collaboration between health care institutions that would compromise a Catholic institution's fidelity to Church teaching. Burke's perspective allows for only a narrow focus on issues that reflect this hierarchy of values, and the common good requires that Catholic health care institutions ensure those values without compromise. He also, however, recognizes a fundamental principle guiding health care: "Catholic teaching on man and conscience in what pertains to health care is found first of all in the Gospel in which an essential and principal part of the public ministry of Christ, God the Son Incarnate, is the care for and healing of the sick."[37] The *ERD* makes a similar assertion in its introduction, focusing on the healing ministry of Christ as the foundational principle of Catholic health care.

There seems to be a tension in both Burke's and the *ERD*s' vision of the common good and how to realize it between the absolute norms prohibiting intrinsically immoral acts and the foundational principle guiding health care. Are these mutually exclusive? Does the common good prohibit certain acts reflected in the Church's absolute norms or does it prioritize the principle of caring for and healing the sick? Does the potential survival of Catholic health care institutions that depend on collaboration with non-Catholic institutions factor into the evaluation of collaborative relationships and the interrelationship between the prioritization of absolute norms and the positive principles and virtues of care, healing, compassion, and mercy? Burke's view attempts to keep Catholic institutions "pure" when such purity may endanger their very survival and their ability to ensure Christ's ministry of healing where their presence is desperately needed.[38]

Cathleen Kaveny asserts that Burke's perspective of the common good is "deeply inadequate," and it is inadequate, we argue, methodologically and anthropologically.[39] Methodologically, it presents both a Manualist act-centered view of the common good and a reductionist view of the social context of Catholic health care. First, for Burke the common good is layered, and we can move to a higher layer only when the foundational layer is fully realized. In the case of collaboration, health care, and the common good, there can be no cooperation unless there is absolute adherence to Church teaching, especially to its absolute norms on sexuality and the end and beginning of life. Second, this act-centered approach is a priori and deductive and does not adequately address a methodological shift toward inductive reasoning and the focus on virtues such as justice, mercy, and compassion illumined by prudence. Third, it fails to realize the complex interrelationships between individuals, groups, and structures, especially structural sin, that impact the interpretation and application of PGC to realize the common good. It prioritizes Catholic sexual teaching and a narrow focus on beginning- and end-of-life issues and ignores multiple other structural issues reflected in Catholic social and environmental teaching. Among those structural issues we list the compensation of CEOs at Catholic and non-Catholic health care institutions, the cost of health care that precludes any preferential option for the poor, and the environmental impacts of health care institutions that may cause or perpetuate illnesses, especially among society's poor and most vulnerable.[40]

Burke's image of the common good and his attempt to maintain institutional purity ignores Pope Francis's challenge to the Church:

> I prefer a Church which is bruised, hurting and dirty because it has been out on the streets, rather than a Church which is unhealthy from being confined and from clinging to its own security. . . . More than by fear of going astray, my hope is that we will be moved by the fear of remaining shut up within structures which give us a false sense of security, within rules which make us harsh judges, within habits which make us feel safe, while at our door people are starving and Jesus does not tire of saying to us: "Give them something to eat" (Mk 6:37). (EG, 49)

It ignores also his challenge to priests to "be shepherds, with the 'odor of the sheep.'"[41] These challenges have both individual and institutional implications.

Individually, priests and all Christians are called to be engaged and to go out and meet people where they are and through accompaniment to be with, minister to, and serve especially the most vulnerable poor. Institutionally, this service of accompaniment ought to be present whenever and wherever Christ's healing ministry is present. This includes Catholic and non-Catholic health care institutions and the collaborative relationships between them. We must not focus on Burke's ideal that prioritizes institutional "purity." We must, rather, embrace Francis's sage Gospel advice to be willing to reflect Christ's healing ministry, even if it means that our "shoes get soiled by the mud of the street" (*AL*, 308) as we cooperate with institutions who practice morally objectionable procedures.

In light of these considerations, we propose a definition of the common good to serve as a hermeneutical lens for interpreting and applying PGC. That definition is informed by Catholic holistic human development and is particular to both individuals and communities and evolving in light of social, cultural, economic, environmental, and structural considerations. The common good must consider the complex interrelationship between individuals, groups, and social structures, competing perspectives of values and meanings, and every attempt to realize the common good through justice, charity, mercy, and compassion aligned with prudence.

Two (or More) Objects

These two perspectives on the common good have implications for how we define the object of the act at the heart of interpreting and applying the principles governing material cooperation. The traditional and manual sources of morality, drawing from Aquinas, teach that the morality of an act involves its object, end, and circumstances in the determination of its morally good or bad quality. Aquinas concluded that all three must be good in order for the act to be morally good. Much ink has been spilled in Catholic theological ethics over whether one can declare certain acts—abortion, contraception, direct sterilization, physician-assisted suicide, euthanasia—intrinsically evil according to their objects alone. For many Catholic ethicists the answer to this question depends on whether one includes the motive for the act in the description of its object. For example, does the use of contraception or direct sterilization necessarily include a contraceptive motive as the Church assumes or can a person choose such acts from a motive of responsible parenthood? Another question is how one defines the object. Is it from the perspective of Church teaching or from the perspective of the acting subject?

In *Veritatis Splendor*, Pope John Paul II asserts that "*the morality of the human act depends primarily and fundamentally on the 'object' rationally chosen by the deliberate will. . . . In order to be able to grasp the object of an act which specifies that act morally,* it is therefore necessary to place oneself *in the perspective of the acting person*" (*VS*, 78, emphasis in original). If one must place oneself in the perspective of the acting person in order to make a moral assessment of an act's object and to determine material cooperation, it seems to be a violation of human dignity and the authority and inviolability of individual conscience to declare certain acts "intrinsically immoral" without consideration of the perspective of the acting person. As we argue in the section on perspectivism, people know and understand in unique ways based on culture, history, context, relationships, and numerous other variables that create different perspectives. Bernard Cooke refers to this as "social location," "the ethnic background, economic situation, educational formation, age and experience, the factors that condition the way people interpret the world around them. People with different social locations see 'reality' quite differently."[42] In our terms, they have different perspectives that allow them to see and interpret the object in ways that may differ from a local bishop's interpretation of the object when considering collaboration. These differences should be discerned and respected through the process of synodality.

The definition of the object and the interrelationship between Catholic moral teaching on individual acts and Catholic social and environmental teaching that emphasizes structures and institutions highlights a point that James Keenan made years ago when reflecting on cooperation in relation to condom use and the prevention of the spread of HIV. There can be at least two competing "objects" with competing values or disvalues when considering PGC. Keenan's article was in reaction to the controversy over the United States Catholic Conference's document, "The Many Faces of AIDS: A Gospel Response." In that document, the conference made a distinction between institutional, structural policies and individual acts, stating that "if grounded in the broader moral vision" institutional educational programs "could include accurate information about prophylactic devices" to stem the spread of HIV. It immediately clarifies that it is "not promoting the use of prophylactics" nor promoting immoral sexual behavior "but merely providing information that is part of the factual [and educational] picture." In the appendix, it notes that individuals who have the virus or who are at risk of contracting it should "live a chaste life."[43] Keenan argues that PGC apply to the United States Catholic Conference document, highlighting the tradition of the principles that focuses on the object of the act to determine the moral nature of cooperation between the cooperator and the wrongdoer. What is the conference's object of cooperation in the document? One object, the institutional emphasis on educational programs about prophylactics, is not promoting immoral sexual behavior but educating the public and protecting the common good by providing information to prevent the spread of HIV. The other object applies to individuals who may use that information "to live a chaste life" or to limit threats to the common good by using prophylactics to prevent the spread of HIV. He summarizes, "by using the prophylactic the object of one's sexual activity remains illicit. The use, however, diminishes the other object of concern, that is, the threat to the common good."[44] Analogously, in collaborative relationships, the harm caused by the individual performance of intrinsically immoral acts at a non-Catholic health care institution may be illicit based on the object of the act, but Christ's healing ministry and the common good are still promoted by such collaborative relationships.

Emphasizing multiple objects in institutional collaboration highlights an important shift in thinking about PGC individually and institutionally. When the principles are applied to institutions, the focus can shift from the evil to be avoided in cooperation to the good that can be achieved in cooperation. This is especially important when addressing institutional cooperation in a pluralistic culture. Following the *ERD*, we maintain that "prioritizing the opportunities to further the mission of Catholic health care" is a primary object and an essential component to realizing the common good. Any challenges that may arise to such cooperation, such as the possibility of institutional scandal, can be dealt with by explaining the role and function of Catholic health care institutions to extend Christ's healing ministry as far as possible, including to non-Catholic institutions.

ERD on Scandal and Witness

The *ERD* insists that any moral analysis of collaboration must take into consideration the possibility of scandal. Cooperation between Catholic and non-Catholic health care institutions that engage in immoral procedures, "even when such cooperation is morally justified in all other respects" (*ERD*, 24), may not be morally permissible if scandal results. Although the *ERD* does not set out a clear hierarchy of criteria for interpreting and applying PGC, the danger of scandal takes precedence in moral analysis since it can trump all other criteria ("justified in all other respects"). We must, then, consider scandal in some detail.

Scandal

The *ERD* draws from the *Catechism* and defines *scandal* as "an attitude or behavior which leads another to do evil" (*ERD*, 24). The *Catechism* continues, "Scandal is a grave offense if by deed or omission another is deliberately led into a grave offense" (*CCC*, 2284), and further, that "anyone who uses the power at his disposal in such a way that it leads others to do wrong becomes guilty of scandal and responsible for the evil that he has directly or indirectly encouraged" (*ERD*, dir. 49; *CCC*, 2287). Causing scandal is a serious moral issue and something to be avoided. What is never clear, however, is how claims of scandal are to be justified. Catholic health care workers should certainly lead by word and example and should be supportive of the teachings of the Catholic Church. Scandal, however, can depend on which teaching of the Catholic Church is emphasized. The *ERD* advances Catholic teaching on "actions that are intrinsically immoral, such as abortion, euthanasia, assisted suicide, and direct sterilization" (dir. 70), but nowhere does it focus on the Catholic teaching on the authority and inviolability of the responsibly informed conscience. Human dignity, the Second Vatican Council teaches, demands the right to follow one's informed conscience (*GS*, 16), and violating the consciences of individual health care workers or of cooperating non-Catholic health care institutions, possibly justifying discrimination against them, might give scandal every bit as much as performing direct sterilization. Scandal, in other words, lies in the eye of the beholder, and, we ask, which claim of scandal is justified in any complex health care moral situation? The assertion that an action would cause scandal is precisely that, an assertion, not a moral argument. Like any other assertion of right or wrong it must be justified by sound moral argument.

The *Catechism* teaches that "the Church's social teaching proposes principles for reflection; it provides criteria for judgment; it gives guidelines for action" (*CCC*, 2423). This trinity—principles for reflection, criteria for judgment, and guidelines for action—is underscored in John Paul II's *Sollicitudo Rei Socialis*. This approach to social morality, an authentically established part of the Catholic moral tradition in modern times, introduces a model of personal responsibility that underscores the responsibility of each person in the communion-synodal Church in any dialogue. John Paul II accentuates this Catholic perspective by teaching that, in its social teachings, the Church seeks "to guide people to respond, with the support of rational reflection and of the human sciences, to their vocation as responsible builders of earthly society" (*SRS*, 1). This teaching applies to any dialogue in a synodal church seeking to responsibly build Catholic health care: church teaching *guides*; responsible believers, drawing on Church guidance, their own experience, attentiveness, understanding, decisiveness, and the findings of the human sciences, *respond*. "Catholic health care should be marked," the *ERD* teaches, "by a spirit of mutual respect among caregivers" (dir. 2), and so should any internal or external dialogue about it. Dialogue about any issue, including health care, should always be characterized by personal freedom, not by the obedience to external authority consistently implied in the *ERD*.

Catholic social teaching and the authority of conscience have several implications for scandal and how to apply it to PGC. First, non-infallible Church teaching contained in directive 70 cannot supersede individual conscience. The *ERD* needs to highlight the authority and inviolability of conscience in relation to its non-infallible norms that prohibit intrinsically immoral acts. This would establish why Catholic health care institutions can cooperate with non-Catholic ones, even with those performing procedures prohibited by Catholic teaching. Second, as discussed in relation to the common good and multiple objects, PGC must evaluate a wide range of harms and benefits, and the *ERD* can provide more specific guidelines for such evaluations. As the *ERD* indicates, the principle of Catholic health care is foundational: Christ's healing ministry. In addition, a central principle of Catholic social teaching is that access to health care is a basic human right and fosters human dignity and the common good.[45] Christ's healing ministry and access to health care are two primary objects that are relevant to any consideration of PGC where the institution's survival or ability to function in health care is at stake or provides an opportunity for Catholic health care to extend this ministry institutionally through non-Catholic health care institutions. Ensuring these two objects by preserving a Catholic health care institution through collaboration with a non-Catholic one can carry as much, and even more, moral weight as any institutional or individual violation of the Church's absolute norms. There are certainly more morally problematic harms, such as those that endanger access to health care or Christ's healing ministry, than cooperation in intrinsically evil acts. An explanation of these two objects and their prioritization in relation to directive 70 to discern PGC could be a helpful addition to the *ERD*. It could help avoid scandal in the eye of the beholder who prioritizes the absolute norms listed in directive 70 over the foundational principles of Catholic health care envisioned by the Catholic Health Association.[46] It could also help to form consciences by promoting a deeper understanding of the benefits of cooperation between Catholic and non-Catholic health care institutions. This deeper understanding would be helpful in assessing the importance of witness as another criterion for considering collaborative relationships.

Witness

The CDF statement begins its response to the USCCB *dubia* by asserting that "from the Church's earliest days, certain Christians, *as part of their prophetic witness to the faith*, have dedicated themselves to the care of the sick."[47] It is clear that the CDF sees witness as a foundational concept of Christian faith and the care for the sick as a clear example of witness. The *ERD* speaks of witness ten times. It is expressed in terms of faith; hope ("the Church witnesses to her belief that God has created each person for eternal life"); love, respect, and support (*ERD*,

20); human dignity ("the sanctity of life 'from the moment of conception until death,'" *ERD*, 16); and "Christ and his Gospel" (*ERD*, 24, 25). The *ERD* paraphrases the CDF's statement on witness in its section on collaboration:

> Even when there are good reasons for establishing collaborative arrangements that involve material cooperation with wrongdoing, leaders of Catholic healthcare institutions must assess whether becoming associated with the wrongdoing of a collaborator will risk undermining their institution's ability to fulfill its mission of providing health care as a *witness* to the Catholic faith and an embodiment of Jesus' concern for the sick. *They must do everything they can to ensure that the integrity of the Church's witness to Christ and his Gospel* is not adversely affected by a collaborative arrangement. (*ERD*, 24; emphasis added)

In all the references to witness, the emphasis is on Jesus' ministry and concern for the sick as an essential component of that ministry. The references to scandal emphasize the violation of natural law, canon law, and Church teaching.[48] An important question for collaboration is to discern the relationship between witness and scandal and how witness is promoted or undermined. Is witness promoted by not entering into, or withdrawing from, collaborative relationships with non-Catholic institutions or, as recommended by Pope Francis (*EG*, 169–73; *AL*, 291ff, 301), by accompanying such institutions and health care workers in a collaborative relationship that promotes cooperation and witness to the Gospel? The USCCB has incorporated into its revised *ERD* neither Francis's teaching on synodality nor his teaching on accompaniment as an aspect of witness. Which is more foundational for Catholic identity and collaborative relationships when assessing the benefits and harms of those relationships? We suggest that witness should be prioritized and promoted through collaborative relationships and the fear of scandal should be confronted to limit or eliminate its risk. The *ERD* prioritizes scandal and the violation of norms that lead others to sin; we prioritize witness as foundational to Catholic identity in health care. Pope Francis's emphasis on accompaniment and smelling like the sheep seems to prioritize witness and Christ's presence in and through healing ministry. An example will illustrate two perspectives on the interpretation and application of the PGC in light of considerations of the common good, conscience, the moral object, scandal, and witness.

COOPERATION: A CASE STUDY

A case that illustrates two different perspectives on the interpretation and application of the PGC to a cooperative relationship is the USCCB's and CHA's respective stances on the accommodation to the so-called contraceptive mandate of the Affordable Care Act.[49] In 2012 the US Department of Health and Human Services announced that it would include various contraceptive services as part of the ACA without charging copays, deductibles, or coinsurance. Previously, in August 2011, HHS approved guidelines that from August 2012 would provide contraception without any additional costs in new health plans. It also announced an exemption clause for religiously affiliated institutions from providing contraceptive services if they fulfilled four criteria. First, they must promote religious values as their purpose; second, they must primarily employ people who share their religious tenets; third, they must primarily serve people who share their religious tenets; and fourth, they must be nonprofit organizations as classified by the Internal Revenue Service code. This religious exemption, however, did not cover most Catholic health care institutions, social services, and education. The final rule of the ACA would take effect in August 2013, and Catholic organizations that did not qualify for the exemption would be required to provide contraceptive services in their insurance plans.

Both the USCCB and the Catholic Health Association strenuously opposed the final rule, arguing that it violated the constitutional protection of religious liberty and the rights of conscience. The White House responded within weeks, announcing an accommodation to the contraceptive mandate. The accommodation allowed religious organizations to fulfill their values by not including, subsidizing, or referring contraceptive services in their insurance plans, and it allowed the HHS and ACA to fulfill its commitment to providing contraceptive services as an essential component of a health care plan. The Catholic Health Association supported the accommodation; the USCCB opposed it, arguing that the mandate should be eliminated.

The conflicting responses to the HHS accommodation by the USCCB and CHA reflect two different perspectives on the criteria guiding the interpretation and application of PGC. The USCCB focused on directive 70 of the *ERD* and on Catholic sexual teaching prohibiting immediate material cooperation in intrinsically immoral actions like contraception. It emphasizes institutional Church conscience over the individual consciences of employees who are among the majority of Catholics who dissent from Catholic sexual teaching on contraception. It prioritizes Catholic sexual teaching's deductive, act-centered, culturally and economically insensitive method. It reflects Cardinal Burke's perspective of a layered vision of the common good, where the prohibition of intrinsically evil acts must be assured before consideration of the benefits of the ACA to millions of uninsured or underinsured people. In Burke's perspective, the benefit of implementing the Church's "social teaching" (*ERD* [2009], 34), the preferential option for the poor, and the realization of health care as a basic human right does not outweigh the harm of providing contraceptive services. The USCCB emphasizes the object of a contraceptive act over the object of universal access to health care. Cardinal Francis George's response to Sister Carol Keehan, CEO of the Catholic Health Association, on health care reform and abortion and Cardinal Timothy Dolan's response to her on the ACA accommodation and the Olmsted case both reflect a hierarchical ecclesiology that emphasizes the bishops' authority and obedience to that authority as a primary virtue.[50] The focus on witness (a later addition in the 2018 *ERD*) seems to be ensuring clarity on the Church's teaching on absolute norms prohibiting contraceptive services. The scandal would be the USCCB's concern that, if there is cooperation with the government and the accommodation, it would risk causing the faithful to be confused about the Church's teachings on contraceptive services and lead them to sin.

The CHA has a different perspective on criteria guiding the interpretation and application of PGC and accommodation. It focuses on Catholic social teaching's preferential option for the poor and access to health care as a basic human right, both of which the ACA seeks to realize. It emphasizes individual conscience over institutional Church conscience, allowing individuals to decide on the basis of an informed conscience whether or not to use contraceptive services in their health plans. It prioritizes Catholic holistic human development over absolute sexual norms and emphasizes an inductive, historically conscious, principle-centered, and culturally and economically sensitive ethical method. The CHA's perspective on the common good reflects a complex reality of social and institutional relationships and structures and promotes its positive goal to realize human fulfillment through access to health care. From this perspective, the benefit of implementing the Church's social teaching—the preferential option for the poor and the realization of health care as a basic human right—outweighs the harm of violating directive 70 and providing contraceptive practices.

The CHA emphasizes the object of universal access to health care and Christ's healing ministry over the object of contraception. It embraces synodality and discernment in its response to the ACA's religious exemption. It reflects the principles of Catholic social teaching and the virtues associated with it as laid out in its proposal for a comprehensive and holistic Catholic model of health care. This model, based on Catholic identity, emphasizes witness as Christ's "healing and reconciling presence to the sick and suffering," providing mercy and hope, a preferential option for the poor, social and environmental justice, and the positive values of a Catholic health care institution rather than avoiding negative disvalues.[51] Any scandal involved would be to risk jeopardizing these foundational values by not cooperating with the ACA and could easily be addressed by explaining Church teaching on PGC, prudential judgment, and contraceptive services that can allow for cooperation. Historically, the USCCB, following Pope John Paul II, has used cooperation for legislators to support laws that limit but do not eliminate abortion.[52] It is curious that it took such a rigid and uncompromising stance against the ACA and its religious exemption from providing contraceptive services. The two different perspectives of the USCCB and the CHA, which lead to conflicting conclusions on the interpretation and application of PGC, highlight that these principles are complex and that good people may disagree on their interpretation and application, depending on their perspectives.

The revised *ERD* takes a cautious tone with respect to collaboration, noting that Catholic health care institutions "should avoid, *whenever possible*, engaging in collaborative arrangements that would involve them in contributing to the wrongdoing of other providers" (*ERD*, 23, emphasis added). It is encouraging to see this more positive approach to collaborative relationships, but the revised *ERD* is still inadequate. It fails to incorporate Pope Francis's anthropological, methodological, and ecclesiological perspectives, especially in light of the sex-abuse scandal, which calls for an ecclesial paradigm shift in how bishops exercise their authority.

SUGGESTED READINGS

Congregation for the Doctrine of the Faith. *Some Principles for Collaboration with Non-Catholic Entities in the Provision of Health Care Services.* Vatican City: Typis Polyglottis Vaticanis, 2014.

Curran, Charles E., ed. *Change in Official Catholic Moral Teachings.* New York: Paulist Press, 2003.

Kaveny, Cathleen. *Law's Virtues: Fostering Autonomy and Solidarity in American Society.* Washington, DC: Georgetown University Press, 2012.

Keenan, James F. "Prophylactics, Toleration, and Cooperation: Contemporary Problems and Traditional Principles." *International Philosophical Quarterly* 29, no. 2 (June 1989): 205–20.

Kelly, David F., Gerard Magill, and Henk Ten Have. *Contemporary Catholic Health Care Ethics.* 2nd ed. Washington, DC: Georgetown University Press, 2013.

Sullivan, Francis A. *Magisterium: Teaching Authority in the Catholic Church.* Dublin: Gill and Macmillan, 1985.

NOTES

1. Ashok Selvam, "Business Conversion," *Modern Healthcare* 42, no. 5 (January 30, 2012): 6–15.

2. Congregation for the Doctrine of the Faith, "Some Principles for Collaboration with Non-Catholic Entities in the Provision of Health Care Services," *National Catholic Bioethics Quarterly* (Summer 2014): 337–40, available at https://www.ncbcenter.org/files/4914/4916/4379/Q14.2_Verbatim_CDF_Principles.pdf.

3. Ethicists of the NCBC, "Introduction to the Sixth Edition," 2.

4. See Gerald A. Arbuckle, *Abuse and Cover-Up: Refounding the Catholic Church in Trauma* (Maryknoll, NY: Orbis, 2019); and Charles Bouchard, OP, "Clergy Sexual Abuse and Catholic Health Care," *Health Progress* (November–December 2019), 19–23, available at https://www.chausa.org/publications/health-progress/article/november-december-2018/clergy-sexual-abuse-and-catholic-health-care.

5. Congregation for the Doctrine of the Faith, "Some Principles," 338.

6. Neil Ormerod, "Sexual Abuse, a Royal Commission, and the Australian Church," *Theological Studies* 80, no. 4 (2019): 950–66, at 963.

7. Bernard J. F. Lonergan, "Dialectic of Authority," in *A Third Collection*, ed. F. Crowe (New York: Paulist, 1985), 3–9; Joseph Komonchak, "Authority and Magisterium," in *Vatican Authority and American Catholic Dissent*, ed. W. May (New York: Crossroad, 1987), 103–14.

8. Lonergan, "Dialectic of Authority," 7–8.

9. Lonergan, 11; Ormerod, "Sexual Abuse," 963–64.

10. Komonchak, "Authority and Magisterium," 107.

11. This is similar to what earlier commentaries on the ERD referred to as a "theology of cooperation." See Commission on Ethical and Religious Directives for Catholic Hospitals, "Catholic Hospital Ethics," *Hospital Progress* 54, no. 2 (February 1973): 44–56, par. 54; and Ron Hamel, "The Ethical and Religious Directives: Looking Back to Move Forward," *Health Progress* (November/December 2019), available at https://www.chausa.org/publications/health-progress/article/november-december-2019/100th-anniversary---the-ethical-and-religious-directives-looking-back-to-move-forward.

12. International Theological Commission, *Synodality in the Life and Mission of the Church* (Vatican City: Libreria Editrice Vaticana, 2018), 38.

13. International Theological Commission, 25.

14. See Leonard Swidler, "Democracy, Dissent, and Dialogue," in *The Church in Anguish*, ed. Hans Kung and Leonard Swidler (San Francisco: Harper & Row, 1986), 306–24, at 310.

15. International Theological Commission, *Synodality in the Life and Mission of the Church*, 64.

16. International Theological Commission, 106.

17. See Henry Davis, *Moral and Pastoral Theology* (London: Sheed and Ward, 1958), 342.

18. Kelly et al., *Contemporary Catholic Health Care Ethics*, 284–85.

19. Ethicists of the NCBC, "Introduction to the Sixth Edition," 3.

20. Robert T. Kennedy, "Chapter II: Juridic Persons," canons 113–23, in *New Commentary on the Code of Canon Law*, ed. John Beal, James Coriden, and Thomas J. Green (New York: Paulist Press, 2000), 154–76, at 154.

21. Kennedy, canons 113, par. 2 and 114.

22. See Francis Morrisey, "Toward Juridic Personality," *Health Progress* (July–August 2001), available at https://www.chausa.org/publications/health-progress/article/july-august-2001/toward-juridic-personality; Charles E. Bouchard, OP, "100th Anniversary: Sponsors Are Called to Be Prophets and Reformers," *Health Progress* (May–June 2019), available at https://www.chausa.org/publications/health-progress/article/may-june-2019/100th-anniversary---sponsors-are-called-to-be-prophets-and-reformers.

23. Cathleen Kaveny, *Law's Virtues: Fostering Autonomy and Solidarity in American Society* (Washington, DC: Georgetown University Press, 2012), 248–49.

24. Kaveny, 249.

25. We are using this phrase euphemistically. As Daniel Finn correctly points out, conscience requires subjectivity, which institutions do not have. In a hierarchical ecclesiology, the institutional conscience is the bishops making decisions "with little or no consultation with others" ("Can an Organization Have a Conscience? Contributions from Social Science to Catholic Social Thought," in *Conscience and Catholicism: Rights, Responsibilities, and Institutional Responses*, ed. David E. DeCosse and Kristin E. Heyer [Maryknoll, NY: Orbis, 2015], 167–81, at 179).

26. Lawrence J. Welch, "Direct Sterilization: An Intrinsically Evil Act—A Rejoinder to Fr. Keenan," *Linacre Quarterly* (May 2001): 124–30, at 124.

27. Welch misrepresents the Catholic tradition on conscience. An amendment was proposed to the Theological Commission at the Second Vatican Council seeking a statement that conscience must be formed "in accord with the doctrine of the Church." The council's Theological Commission rejected the proposal as "unduly restrictive." See Second Vatican Council, *Acta Synodalia* (Vatican City: Typis Polyglottis Vaticanis, 1970), IV/6, 769.

28. Canon Law Society of America, *Code of Canon Law, Latin-English Edition* (Washington, DC: Canon Law Society of America, 1983).

29. Canon Law Society of America, *Code of Canon Law, Latin-English Edition: New English Translation* (Washington, DC: Canon Law Society of America, 1999).

30. Francis A. Sullivan, *Magisterium: Teaching Authority in the Catholic Church* (Dublin: Gill and Macmillan, 1985), 164. See also James A. Coriden, "Introduction," in *New Commentary on the Code of Canon Law*, who argues that "an exact translation of *obsequium* is difficult but 'submission' is not the best one because it exaggerates the force of the Latin" (916).

31. See Curran, *Change in Official Catholic Moral Teachings*; John T. Noonan, *A Church That Can and Cannot Change* (Notre Dame, IN: University of Notre Dame Press, 2005).

32. James A. Coriden, Thomas J. Green, and Donald E. Heintschel, eds., *The Code of Canon Law: A Text and Commentary* (New York: Paulist, 1985), 548.

33. See Todd A. Salzman and Michael G. Lawler, "*Amoris Laetitia* and the Development of Catholic Theological Ethics: A Reflection," in *A Point of No Return?* Amoris Laetitia *on Marriage, Divorce and Remarriage*, ed. Thomas Knieps (Münster: Verlag, 2017), 30–44.

34. See Hamel, "Ethical and Religious Directives."

35. See Cardinal Raymond Burke, "Keynote Address, National Catholic Prayer Breakfast," LifeSiteNews.com, May 8, 2009, available at https://mariancatechist.com/wp-content/uploads/2019/02/abpburkencpbkeynote2009.pdf; Welch, "Direct Sterilization."

36. Cardinal Raymond Burke, "The Economy of Life and the Catholic Identity of Catholic Hospitals in an Age of Secularization," *Linacre Quarterly* 85, no. 2 (May 2018): 106–14, available at https://www.ncbi.nlm.nih.gov/pmc/articles/PMC6056805/.

37. Burke.

38. See James Keenan, "Institutional Cooperation and the Ethical and Religious Directives," *Linacre Quarterly* 64, no. 3 (August 1997): 53–76, at 65, for an example of the ethical costs of attempting to maintain such purity in Catholic university health care facilities.

39. Kaveny, *Law's Virtues*, 258.

40. See Michael Rozier, "Collective Action on Determinants of Health: A Catholic Contribution," *Health Progress* (September/October 2019): 5–8; Howard Gleckman, "Social

Determinants of Health: Moving beyond the Buzzwords," *Health Progress* (July–August 2019): 76–77; Nathaniel Blanton Hibner, "How Should Health Care Respond to Social Challenges?" *Health Progress* (March–April 2019): 63–64. See Hamel, "Ethical and Religious Directives," 69.

41. "Homily of Pope Francis," March 28, 2013, available at http://www.vatican.va/content/francesco/en/homilies/2013/documents/papa-francesco_20130328_messa-crismale.html.

42. Bernard Cooke, "Winds of Change Bring a 'Paradigm Shift': Now Faithful Must Speak Up," *National Catholic Reporter*, June 7, 2013, https://www.ncronline.org/news/theology/winds-change-bring-paradigm-shift-now-faithful-must-speak.

43. NCCB, "The Many Faces of Aids: A Gospel Response" (Washington, DC: NCCB, 1987), available at http://www.usccb.org/issues-and-action/human-life-and-dignity/global-issues/statement-the-many-faces-of-aids-from-nccb-administrative-board-1987-11.cfm.

44. James F. Keenan, "Prophylactics, Toleration, and Cooperation: Contemporary Problems and Traditional Principles," *International Philosophical Quarterly* 29, no. 2 (June 1989): 206–20, at 212.

45. See USCCB, "Joint Letter to Congress: ACA Principles," March 8, 2017, available at http://www.usccb.org/issues-and-action/human-life-and-dignity/health-care/upload/Joint-Letter-to-Congress-ACA-Principles-03-07-2017.pdf.

46. Catholic Health Association of the United States, "Our Vision for U.S. Health Care" (2019), available at https://www.chausa.org/docs/default-source/advocacy/cha_2019_visionforushealthcare_080819-singles.pdf.

47. CDF, "Some Principles," 337, emphasis added.

48. See Hayley Penan and Amy Chen, "The Ethical and Religious Directives: What the 2018 Update Means for Catholic Hospital Mergers," *National Health Law Program* (January 2, 2019), available at https://healthlaw.org/resource/the-ethical-religious-directives-what-the-2018-update-means-for-catholic-hospital-mergers/.

49. See Kelly et al., *Contemporary Catholic Health Care Ethics*, 280–84.

50. "Church Leaders Diverge on Reform: C.H.A. Accepts Senate Language," *America*, March 29, 2010, available at https://www.americamagazine.org/issue/731/signs/church-leaders-diverge-reform-cha-accepts-senate-language; Kevin Clarke, "CHA and USCCB: Making Up Is Hard to Do?" *America*, February 1, 2011, available at https://www.americamagazine.org/content/all-things/cha-and-usccb-making-hard-do.

51. Michael R. Panicola and Ron Hamel, "Catholic Identity and Reshaping of Health Care in the United States," *Health Progress*, July 24, 2015, available at https://www.chausa.org/publications/health-care-ethics-usa/archives/issues/summer-2015/catholic-identity-and-the-reshaping-of-health-care-in-the-united-states.

52. USCCB, *Forming Consciences for Faithful Citizenship: A Call to Political Responsibility from the Catholic Bishops of the United States* (Washington, DC: USCCB, 2009), 32, available at http://www.usccb.org/issues-and-action/faithful-citizenship/upload/forming-consciences-for-faithful-citizenship.pdf. See John Paul II, *Evangelium Vitae*, 73.

CHAPTER SEVEN

Suggestions for a Revised *ERD*

In the conclusion to his 1984 commentary on the *ERD*, Richard McCormick explains that health care ethics is in a state of transition that includes both "coming from" and "going forward." The past is alive and must inform the discipline as it moves forward. He is optimistic that moving forward in health care ethics will reflect the collegiality, collaboration, and, in Pope Francis's word, synodality that marked the pastoral letters "The Challenge of Peace" and "Economic Justice for All." These pastoral letters of the American Catholic bishops in consultation with theologians and lay experts in the field highlight a communion ecclesiology in the consideration of peace, war, and economic justice. They were creative, hopeful, firmly grounded theologically, ethically, anthropologically, and methodologically. They inspired hope in episcopal leadership, vision, and incarnation of a communion church, and they inspired a profound trust in lay people, priests, theologians, economists, and ethicists, who discerned in them concrete and hopeful responses to complex issues in light of the signs of the times. Reflecting on health care ethics, McCormick anticipates that such vision, leadership, and collegiality will continue: "There must and will be more collegiality in the establishment of policy for health care institutions."[1]

McCormick's vision and hope for "going forward" has not yet come to fruition, and there are several reasons for this. First, there has been a growing polarization in the Church, which leads to suspicion and distrust between bishops, progressive theologians, and laity. In hierarchical, clerical, and patriarchal institutions that view themselves under threat, real or imagined, from social, cultural, and political assaults on religious liberty, a common response is to reassert power and authority in an attempt to reestablish the perception that the institution is stable and flourishing rather than in turmoil and risking irrelevance. The sociological data do not lie: a high percentage of Catholics disagree with absolute Catholic norms on sexual and health care ethical issues. Nones, those who have no religious affiliation, are the second-largest religious group in the United States at 23.1 percent of the population, and former Catholics make up a large part of the nones. The Catholic percentage of the adult population in the United States has dropped from 23 percent in 2009 to 20 percent in 2019, and many of those who consider themselves Catholic judge bishops and their statements on ethical issues as lacking credibility or simply irrelevant. The sex-abuse crisis has further diminished bishops' moral authority and credibility, and the data indicate that the majority of the laity take no stock in bishops' attempt to reassert their authority in the *ERD*.[2]

A second major factor that has led to the loss of episcopal authority and credibility is the sex-abuse crisis. The main factor that forced the bishops to address the sex-abuse crisis in 2002 with the publication of the Dallas Charter was the *Boston Globe*'s Spotlight, which exposed the extent of clerical sexual abuse and its episcopal cover-up. The bishops' response in Dallas was not driven primarily by concern for the children who were sexually abused by some priests and bishops. They went to great lengths to cover up this abuse by moving predatory priests to other parishes, fighting allegations of clerical sexual abuse with high-paid attorneys, and paying out settlements to abused victims with nondisclosure clauses that prevented victims from speaking out. The bishops in Dallas responded, quite simply, because they got caught and their misdeeds were exposed. This crisis has fundamentally transformed public perceptions of bishops individually and collectively, and the USCCB appears to remain deaf to the damage it has caused. As a body it continues to act as if its authority and credibility remain intact, as if people will continue to conform to its dictates. While many laity have moved beyond a hierarchical, clerical model of Church, many bishops have not, and many Catholics have left the Church and moved into the category of nones, giving up on the Church's leadership.

Third, Pope Francis has made monumental strides in renewing the Church and its central message of compassionate and merciful partner-accompanying people on a journey toward Christian discipleship in the contemporary world. The USCCB, unfortunately, has not embraced Francis's ecclesiological vision of synodality, anthropological vision of holistic human dignity, or methodological vision of new pastoral and ethical methods. The revised *ERD* demonstrates that the USCCB lacks the courage, the vision, and the leadership reflected in the pastoral letters on peace and the economy and is far from enhancing McCormick's vision of transition from a classicist, static worldview to a historically conscious, dynamic worldview. Instead, it looks backward, seeking to reestablish a Church that lacks the ecclesial and moral vision of the Second

Vatican Council. It has resisted Pope Francis's holistic anthropology and ethical methodology that seeks truth through synodality, his emphasis on care for the poor, and his concern for environmental justice. In his recent exhortation following the Amazon Synod, *Querida Amazonía*, even Pope Francis seems to have backed away from his own ecclesial and ethical vision under pressure from conservative bishops.[3] He decided to ignore the majority recommendation of the bishops of Amazonia for a married priesthood and women deacons in regions in Amazonia that lack priests and access to the sacraments. This unfortunate decision appears to be the result of an entrenched and vocal minority of bishops who resist reading the signs of the times and responding with trust in the Holy Spirit working in the Church to transition it to relevance in a pluralistic cultural context in need of Christ's sacramental and healing presence. This same conservative worldview is driving many decisions and documents issued by the USCCB, including the revised *ERD*.

Throughout this commentary we have highlighted tensions in the revised *ERD* between its doctrinal and ethical teaching and the dominant doctrine and ethics in the contemporary Catholic theological and ethical community. In this final chapter, we summarize the anthropological, methodological, ecclesiological, pastoral/spiritual, and collaborative tensions within the *ERD* and propose guidelines for an authentic transition in Catholic health care in general and the *ERD* in particular.

ANTHROPOLOGICAL TENSIONS

We have noted several times that the ethical good in Catholic teaching is human dignity. There are, however, different perspectives in the Church on human dignity and, therefore, also different definitions of human dignity. In chapter 2 we dealt with the two major ones, Catholic sexual human dignity and Catholic social human dignity, both of which weave in and out of the *ERD*. We proposed a third definition, which is an integration of those two and which we called Catholic holistic human dignity. Here we further reflect on Catholic sexual and holistic human dignity, especially as they affect Catholic health care ethics.

Relying on his biblical exegesis of Genesis and the teaching of his predecessors, especially on Pope Paul VI's encyclical *Humanae Vitae*, Pope John Paul II developed a comprehensive definition of Catholic sexual human dignity, what he labels a personalist anthropology. This personalist anthropology, and the Church teaching now based on it, is a good example of how terminology can change, from human nature to human person, for instance, and still carry traditional conceptual and terminological baggage. John Paul's works are laden with references to the person, personal dignity, and personal responsibility, but these references are frequently explained and defined in terms of abstract nature and more often than not ignore the concrete human, relational experience of married couples.[4] He notes that "in the order of love a man can remain true to the person only in so far as he is true to nature. If he does violence to 'nature' he also 'violates' the person by making it an object of enjoyment rather than an object of love." Contraception is a violation of nature, and it has a "damaging effect on love."[5] Love and procreation are intrinsically linked in John Paul's theology of the body and Church teaching on complementarity, but in this relationship there is a clear hierarchy of the physical over the personal and relational.[6]

Personalism, we argue, should embrace a holistic understanding of historical human persons in all their biological, psychological, relational, and spiritual complexity. If this is true, then the biological and physical is only one dimension of the human person, indeed a lower dimension subject to the higher dimensions of the person, and should not be given the inordinate importance assigned to it as the primary foundation for human sexual anthropology and dignity. Authentic personalism takes historical persons in the concrete personal, embodied, relational complexity given to them by the creator God and formulates normative guidelines for sexual relationships on a profound appreciation of that complexity. John Paul II's and the Church's notion of complementarity lacks an appreciation and integration for the whole human person, biologically, psychologically, relationally, and spiritually. To the extent that the *ERD* and its directives are based on John Paul II's Catholic sexual human dignity in addressing sexual ethical issues such as contraceptives (*ERD*, 16, dir. 52) and reproductive technologies (*ERD*, 17, dir. 38, 39, 41), it also lacks this appreciation and integration for the whole concrete person. John Paul's sexual human dignity (founded as it is on heterogenital, biological complementarity) requires a more holistic perspective.[7] Pope Francis's *Amoris Laetitia* provides such a perspective.

In his apostolic exhortation *Amoris Laetitia*, his response to two synods on the family, Pope Francis achieves an integration and expansion of Catholic sexual and social human dignity, which we have called Catholic holistic human dignity. *Amoris Laetitia*, for instance, recognizes the impact poverty has on human relationships and ethical decisions. Francis offers an example of a couple who cohabit "primarily because celebrating a marriage is considered too expensive in the social circumstances. As a result, material poverty drives people into de facto unions" (*AL*, 294). He does not focus on these unions as a violation of the absolute norms prohibiting cohabitation and fornication. Rather, following Catholic social teaching, he acknowledges that socioeconomic realities profoundly impact concrete human relationships, judgments, and decisions and that this impact is often overlooked in Church teaching, as it is in the *ERD* that proposes one-size-fits-all norms in its prioritization of the biological and pro-creative over the relational in Catholic sexual human dignity. Francis focuses on relationship and the need to offer cohabiting couples "a constructive response seeking to transform them into opportunities that can lead to the full reality of marriage and family in conformity with the Gospel" (*AL*, 294). Pietro Cardinal Parolin, the Vatican's secretary of state, judges that this ethical approach indi-cates a "paradigm shift" that calls for a "new spirit, a new [method]" to help "incarnate the Gospel in the family."[8] In its most recent edition of the *ERD*, the conservative-leaning USCCB has not demonstrated any awareness, or inclusion, of this ethical paradigm shift.

Pope Francis's *Amoris Laetitia* is in pacific continuity with anthropological developments in both Catholic social and sexual human dignity and expands on those developments by emphasizing a person's capacity for conscience, dis-cernment, and virtue. It also more thoroughly integrates the methods of Cath-olic social and sexual teaching. These developments indicate the need for the revision of some Catholic sexual norms and directives that we have already addressed. *Amoris Laetitia* presents Francis's holistic sexual human dignity and sexual anthropology that draw from the relational emphasis in Catholic social human dignity and a relationally focused personalist anthropology in Cath-olic sexual human dignity. In its absolute proscriptive norms, John Paul II's Catholic sexual human dignity, and the *ERD* that follows him, prioritizes the biological and procreative function of the sexual act over its profound relational meanings. Pope Francis emphasizes the relational and spiritual in every ethical decision, whether it be a decision about a sexual issue or a health care issue. This is especially evident in his emphasis on new pastoral methods and personal conscience that we dealt with at length. We have no doubt that Francis's model of Catholic holistic human dignity is both more faithful to the long-established Catholic tradition on the authority and inviolability of personal conscience and more attuned to the ethical and health care issues of women and men in the third millennium.

METHODOLOGICAL TENSIONS

Catholic social teaching is principle focused, inductive, and historically con-scious. Catholic sexual teaching teaches absolute norms and is act focused, deductive, and classicist when addressing ethical issues at the beginning and end of life. There are clear tensions in the *ERD* between the methods of Catholic social, sexual, and health care teachings guiding the formulation, justification, interpretation, and application of its directives. All three teachings are detectable in the *ERD* as we demonstrate in chapter 3.

To guide the revision of the *ERD*, we propose Pope Francis's recent work in *Amoris Laetitia*, which proposes "new pastoral methods," and in *Laudato Si'*, both of which contribute methodological considerations to Catholic health care teaching by investigating the reciprocal relationship between environmental and social ethics and how they impact health care, including sexual, ethical teaching. Francis's development of integral ecology in *Laudato Si'* complements his new pastoral methods recommended in *Amoris Laetitia* and has profound implications for developing an ecological health care ethics. Focusing on the virtue of care, *Laudato Si'* addresses the need to protect and preserve vital values, especially the human dignity of the poor, who suffer the most from any environmental damage. The virtue of care is a central virtue for ecological ethics and Christ's healing ministry in health care ethics. The two assaults on vital human values, climate change and environmental pollution, cause numerous health hazards and millions of premature deaths across the world (*LS*, 20), especially among the world's poor. *Laudato Si'* also highlights another vital value, the interdependence of all creation: "Because all creatures are connected, each must be cherished with love and respect, for all of us as living creatures are dependent on one another" (*LS*, 42).

Pope Francis's new pastoral methods in *Amoris Laetitia* and ecological ethics in *Laudato Si'* call for greater methodological integration of Catholic social, ecological, sexual, and health care teachings. An essential methodological consideration in both *Amoris Laetitia* and *Laudato Si'* that brings together these teachings and has implications for Catholic health care teaching is the recognition of worldwide poverty and its profound impact on ethical decisions. Socioeconomic and environmental realities profoundly impact human relationships, and these impacts are often overlooked in Church health care teaching that proposes norms that are one-size-fits-all.

The integration of Catholic social, environmental, and sexual ethics also has profound implications for how we formulate and justify norms and directives to guide conscience and how we navigate disagreements between Church teaching and informed consciences in Catholic health care institutions. First, it is the role and inviolable authority of conscience to determine whether or not a norm has anything to say about a particular life situation. The teaching of *Dignitatis Humanae* cannot be doubted: "In all his activity [therefore in all decisions, medical and pastoral, about his health care] a man is bound to follow his conscience faithfully, in order that he may come to God for whom he was created. It follows that he is not to be forced to act contrary to his conscience. Nor, on the other hand, is he to be restrained from acting according to his conscience, especially in matters religious" (*DH*, 3). An informed conscience, the decision made after considering all the relevant factors that I must do this action rather than that one, is the ultimate moral decision-maker and is inviolable.

Second, this emphasis on the authority of conscience must respect the consciences of both health care professionals who are treating patients and patients who are being treated. In the current *ERD*, the local bishop's authority usurps and trumps both the patient's and the health care professional's consciences in the interpretation and application of the *ERD*. This is a clear violation of conscience ethically, methodologically, and ecclesiologically: "The patient is the primary decisionmaker in all choices regarding health and treatment. This means that he or she is the first decisionmaker, the one who is presumed to make initial choices, based on his or her beliefs and values." Health care professionals are "secondary decisionmakers, with responsibility to provide aid and care for the patient to the extent it is consistent with their own beliefs and values."[9] Health care professionals should help patients to inform their consciences with sufficient and accurate medical information to enable the patient to make an informed choice. If the patient's decision of conscience conflicts with that of health care professionals, then an ethics committee should review the decision and make a recommendation. The bishop can and ought to participate in this process, but he should not have the final say on any medical treatment. The medical institution, too, must retain autonomy following best practices for health care. The Phoenix case clearly demonstrates a bishop's violation of the consciences of both an individual patient and health care professionals, as well as of best medical practice. Such decision-making authority by a bishop that usurps consciences and institutional autonomy is, unfortunately, justified by the *ERD* and reflects the ecclesiological tensions in it.

ECCLESIOLOGICAL TENSIONS

In chapter 4 we spoke of ecclesiological tensions in the *ERD* between two models of Church, a hierarchical model, which dominated Catholic thinking prior to the Second Vatican Council and is still prominent in the *ERD*, and a synodal-communion model, overwhelmingly approved as a preferred model of Church by that council and confirmed and developed in Pope Francis's papacy. A major ecclesiological tension in the revised *ERD* is its preference for the hierarchical model, as if it were still 1910 rather than 2020. It insistently highlights the unquestioned authority of the local bishop in Catholic health care because of his ecclesiastical office, not his competence: "The ultimate responsibility for the interpretation and application of the Directives rests with the diocesan Bishop" (*ERD*, 25). He "exercises responsibilities that are rooted in his office [not his competence] as pastor, teacher, and priest." In the absence of any determination by the magisterium, he is the one to determine "approved authors" for guidance in moral questions (*ERD*, 7). This is clearly a hierarchical approach in tension with the synodal-communion model that is the preferred contemporary Catholic model of Church.

The tension is not located in the fact that it is a hierarchical approach, for bishops retain legitimate authority in the communion model. The tension is found, rather, in the fact that it completely ignores the implications of the communion model in which all believers share common responsibility for the common good, including the good of health care. This is nowhere more obvious in the *ERD* than in its suggestion that the local bishop seek the moral guidance of only "approved authors" (*ERD*, 7), usually authors selected by him because they agree with his preformed magisterial judgments. A communion or synodal approach would seek the guidance of all who are competent in the matter, clerical and lay, those who agree or disagree with the bishop, who can in concert offer broader and appropriate guidance in health care issues. This synodal process was initiated by the Catholic Health Association in 1998 to gain clarity in the interpretation and application of the principle of cooperation.[10] Participating members included theologians of different perspectives from academia, the church and health care, and several bishops. However, many of the insights and recommendations of that committee were not incorporated into the *ERD*, and the synodal ecclesiology it represented has been abandoned in favor of the bishop's authority in consultation with approved authors. This is another indication that the hierarchical model continues to dominate in the *ERD*.

PASTORAL TENSIONS

Pope Francis's new pastoral methods have profound implications for the *ERD* methodologically, anthropologically, and pastorally. In chapter 5, we dealt with the *ERD*'s section "Pastoral and Spiritual Responsibility of Catholic Health Care." Catholic teaching about the origin and constitution of the human being continues to be firm: the human is created in the image of God (Gen. 1:26) and is composed of body and soul. That teaching founds the dignity of human beings as not only physical but also, perhaps especially, spiritual beings destined for a life with God, both in their present history and when that history has ended in physical death. The spiritual dignity of human animals makes them different from every other animal; it demands from them a spiritual life beyond the physical and demands from those who minister to them assistance with this spiritual life. The Catholic Church seeks to respond to this demand for spiritual life in its ministry, particularly its liturgical ministry. Humans need that spiritual ministry most when their historical lives, and, therefore, also their spiritual lives, are in any way threatened, and that is the situation with people who are ill and especially those who are dying. Catholic health care has the responsibility to treat those who are ill or dying in a way that respects not only their physical but also their spiritual lives (*ERD*, 10). It has the responsibility to care not only for physical illness but also for spiritual persons. In the *ERD*, that responsibility does not seem to extend beyond the administration of sacraments, which in our experience when hospitalized in a Catholic hospital was a very perfunctory administration far removed from any suggestion of spirituality. Yet the emphasis in Catholic health care ethics is Christ's sacramental healing ministry as a living symbol through the care, mercy, compassion, and presence of all health care professionals, including pastoral ministers.

The *ERD* offers no definition of spiritual health care, perhaps because the Catholic meaning of *spiritual* and *spirituality* has altered over the years and the definition is now contested. In the not-too-distant past, the word *spiritual* was reserved for the minority of monks and nuns who were striving to be perfectly spiritual by living a rigorous lifestyle and a disciplined prayer life withdrawn from the world. That situation has changed, and those who are called nones, the second-largest "religious" group in the United States, often describe themselves as not *religious*, not following an institutional life of prayer and sacrament, but still deeply *spiritual* and introspective into the depth of their lives. The keynote of Catholic spirituality is holistic human experience. Schneiders defines it as "the experience of conscious involvement in the project of life integration through self-transcendence toward the ultimate value one perceives. It is an effort to bring all of life together in an integrated synthesis of ongoing growth and development."[11] It embraces the whole life of every person—soul, body, relationships, religion—and in its Catholic manifestation, we insist, it embraces specifically the presence of God embedded in the depth of that life and experience and waiting to be discovered. Catholics live spiritual lives, we argue, when they acknowledge in faith the presence of God indwelling both them and the world in which they live, and when they respond to that presence of God in the ordinariness of their daily lives. It is a major task of Catholic pastoral care to illuminate the continuing presence and gracious action of God in times of illness and when facing physical death and to nurture a response in faith to that presence and action.

The approach to spirituality and health care we have adopted and recommend is influenced by a 2008 report from the World Health Organization that distinguishes and contrasts what we will call the disease-control model of health care and the person-centered model of health care.[12] The former focuses on *disease* in persons, the latter focuses on *persons who are diseased*. In the disease-control model, the relationship between a sick person and health care professionals ends when the disease is cured; in the person-centered model, it continues as person-centered care in a community. In the disease-control model, health care professionals are responsible for disease control in both individual persons and communities; in the person-centered model, persons are responsible for their own health and that of their community. Given that the mission of Catholic health care is rooted in the Christ-healer who "came that they may have life and have it more abundantly" (John 10:10; *ERD*, 6), the person-centered model of health care appears to us as the more Catholic model. We are fully aware that the dominant model presently is the disease-control model and that it will take a serious sea change in the health care communities to supplant it with a person-centered model. There are some encouraging signs, however, in the person-centered training of physicians, nurses, and other health care professionals, and some also in the training of pastoral and spiritual care professionals.

There is an analogy for the difficult transition from the physically based disease-control model of health care to the holistic person-centered model in the equally difficult Catholic transition from the physically based procreative-institution model of marriage to the holistic interpersonal-union model (see *ERD*, 16, dirs. 52 and 53). After the inhuman horrors of the First World War, when millions of persons were senselessly slaughtered, a philosophical move-ment known as *personalism* developed in Europe and eventually exercised an in-fluence on Catholic theology. The German theologian Dietrich von Hildebrand applied this personalism to marriage. The modern age (his 1930s but still true in the 2000s), he argued, is guilty of an anti-personalism, a blindness toward the dignity of the spiritual person. This blindness is expressed in what he called biological materialism, in which "human life is considered exclusively from a biological point of view and biological principles are the measure by which all human activities are judged."[13] The Catholic Church's procreative-institution model of marriage, with its focus on bodies and their biological functions, is wide open to this charge of biological materialism, and so too is the disease-control model of health care. Both ignore the higher, personal, and spiritual characteristics of the human person. A 2013 Pew Research Poll found that 76 percent of American Catholics do not follow the Church's procreative-institution model of marriage, and we have no doubt that with committed and concerted effort the same thing can happen with the disease-control model of health care in Catholic health care settings.

The disease model is clearly evident in the Catholic sexual teaching that allows the use of contraceptives to treat a physical pathology but prohibits their use in a marriage in which natural family planning to regulate fertility is creating stress and tension between the spouses. The same biologism is evident in the recent statement by the Congregation for Catholic Education, "Male and Female He Created Them." In the case of intersex people, people born with ambiguously gendered reproductive organs, "Male and Female He Created Them" asserts that it is a physician's task to determine the most appropriate therapeutic ends to establish in the least biologically invasive manner possible a person's "constitutive identity," or biological sex. The magisterium has never explicitly condemned sex reassignment surgery, but it has condemned "transsexual surgery," arguing that "the physical integrity of a person cannot be impaired to cure an illness of psychic or spiritual origin. . . . It is different with psychic sufferings and spiritual disorders with an organic [biological] basis, that is, which arise from a defect or physical disease: on these it is legitimate to intervene therapeutically."[14] In the case of an intersex person, where there is an organic origin of what are judged to be "ambiguous genitalia," physician-determined intervention can be used to bring the person's reproductive organs in line with expectations for either male or female identity. In the case of transgender persons, for whose condition "Male and Female He Created Them" assumes a psychic or spiritual origin, no such therapeutic intervention is justified. A biological or physical source warrants medical intervention; a psychic or spiritual source does not.

This attempt to distinguish between the physical and psychic in the case of health care and to reduce health care to a biological, disease-control model rather than a holistic, relational, person-centered model is problematic for several reasons. First, the bifurcation of the physical and psychic dimensions of the person reflects a dualistic anthropology that fails to recognize the profound unity of body and psyche. The medical community well knows that the physical origins of an illness can cause serious psychic illnesses such as depression, suicidal thoughts, and inability to relate to others, and that the mental origins of an illness like stress can cause physical illnesses such as diabetes, Alzheimer's, heart disease, and gastrointestinal issues. What is the causal relationship between physical and psychic illnesses, and why is one privileged over the other when considering therapeutic interventions? A physical pathology, or perceived gender ambiguity in the case of intersex children, that may cause psychic suffering may warrant medical intervention; a psychic origin in the case of marital distress caused by practicing natural family planning that causes the spouses psychic suffering does not warrant such intervention. The inconsistency is attributable to a biology-prioritized anthropology; a holistic-relational anthropology would recognize both physical and psychic origins of suffering as ethical justification for treatment. Second, there is an implicit biological bias in the assertion that physical illness is "more real" than psychic illness.[15] Psychic illness is just as real as, and sometimes more devastating than, physical illness for the health and flourishing of individuals. The *ERD* must overcome a dualistic anthropology, grounded in a biological ontology, both pastorally and medically.

What is natural or unnatural for human animals who are persons is not to be decided on the basis of what is natural or unnatural for non-human animals. Persons are specifically spiritual animals, vitalized by a spiritual soul, and they ought not to be judged exclusively on the basis of barnyard animal biology. Persons are essentially free and inviolable subjects and ought never to be treated as objects. They are also essentially subjects in relation, with self, with other human subjects called neighbors, and ultimately with God. This brings us back to Schneiders's reworked definition of spirituality: "the experience of conscious involvement in the project of life integration through [self-discovery and] self-transcendence toward the ultimate value one perceives."

The keynote of contemporary Catholic spirituality, we have argued, is *experience*, the experience of human life consciously reflected on. The Second Vatican Council's *Gaudium et Spes* emphasized this in 1964, explaining that it would consider a number of urgent needs of the contemporary world "in the light of the gospel and of *human experience*" (*GS*, 46). Contemporary Catholic spirituality is about reading not only the gospels but also the simple and complex experience that people share every day. That experience is sometimes a sinful experience that obscures the presence of God in human life, but it is never an experience that can totally eliminate that presence, even in serious illness, for the gift of God's presence to God's creatures, once given, is never retracted. It remains constant, obscured maybe, but always there waiting to be discovered or rediscovered. The Catholic spiritual tradition has long-established methods for uncovering the presence of God in human experience, introspection, meditation, contemplation, long thought to be methods exclusive to monks and nuns but now available to all who wish to seek the presence of God in this life to sustain them unto the next. Given the experience of illness, we believe we can safely say that the discovery of the presence of God is never more necessary for humans than when they are ill and facing death, and it is the mission of Catholic pastoral care to help the sick and dying to find the comfort and the strength and the joy of the presence of the gracious God in their lives, even when they are ill and dying.

The revised *ERD* recognizes that "pastoral care is an integral part of Catholic health care" and describes it as encompassing "the full range of spiritual services, including a listening presence; help in dealing with powerlessness, pain and alienation; and assistance in recognizing and responding to God's will with greater joy and peace" (*ERD*, 10). We parse "God's will" for the sick and the dying to mean, as it does for all women and men, that they recognize and respond to God's presence in their lives. It is that recognition and response that brings the joy and peace the *ERD* speaks of. In the disease-control model of health care, Catholic pastoral care was consistently interpreted as prayer and administration of sacraments, and the *ERD* retains a commitment to this approach (dirs. 12, 13, 14, 15, 16). We make one proviso about that approach: opportunities for participating in sacramental life should indeed be offered to the sick, but they should be offered in a thoroughly person-centered way, not mechanistically as was often the case in the past. One day after major heart surgery and still in a fog from the anesthetic, a voice instructed me out of the fog to "open your mouth" and, when I obeyed and unreflectingly opened my mouth, Eucharist was with difficulty inserted into it. Hardly the most personal or rewarding way to communicate with the Lord. The *ERD*, we believe, seeks to eliminate such mechanical procedures by specifically demanding "a listening presence" in Catholic pastoral health care, pointing with this phrase to a person-centered health care model. The listening presence of a pastoral minister will hear the concerns, anxieties, and fears of the sick or dying person, respond to them by assisting her to discern the presence and multiple graces of God in her sick life, and lead her to a Christian peace and joy in her sickness or perhaps imminent death.

It is obvious that a person-centered approach to pastoral health care is time consuming and cannot be fully achieved in what today are most often short hospital stays. That, however, is not an argument against the person-centered approach but an argument for greater personal commitment and creativity from the Catholic community for the health not only of this individual sick person but also of the whole community. We have pointed out two important differences between the disease-control and the person-centered models of health care. In the former, the relationship between a sick person and health care professionals ends when the disease is cured; in the person-centered model, it continues as person-centered pastoral care in the Catholic community. In the disease-control model, health care professionals are responsible for disease control in both individual persons and populations; in the person-centered model, persons are responsible, in cooperation with health care professionals, for their own health and for the common good of their community.

The sick person is in control of the treatment for her disease to the extent that either she or her designated representative for health care is free to decide what may or may not be done to her medically, and she is in full control of her search for personal health. If and when she leaves a medical facility on completion of her clinical treatment, she can still continue her search for personal health in a Catholic pastoral care center. Every diocese should have one staffed by competent professionals to which people who are in ill health can go, before possible hospitalization or after release from the hospital, for guided discernment of the presence and grace of God in their challenged lives. The many drug rehabilitation centers already in existence are good models for the pastoral care facilities we have in mind. We fully understand that such centers will cost economically, but the cost pales in comparison to the benefits to both the personal and common good. Catholics, we suggest, especially wealthy Catholics, regularly contribute large sums of money to less worthy, and self-serving, political causes.

The *ERD* asserts that "the biblical mandate to care for the poor requires us to express this in concrete actions at all levels of Catholic health care" (*ERD*, 8), and we agree. It goes on to define those whom it understands to be among the poor and vulnerable: "the [economically] poor; the uninsured and underinsured; children and the unborn; single parents; the elderly; those with incurable diseases and chemical dependencies; racial minorities; immigrants and refugees" (dir. 3). Many of those poor are unhealthy poor, as the COVID-19 pandemic has tragically demonstrated, and we believe the *ERD* either simply forgot or felt there was no need to specify the correlation between poverty and its impact on health. Jesus, whom Christians confess as the Christ, was a notable healer, and the gospels draw special attention to his acts of healing. They show that he did not heal only physical afflictions but "touched people at the deepest level of their existence; he sought their physical, mental and spiritual healing (John 6:35; 11:25–27). He 'came that they may have life and have it more abundantly'" (John 10:10; *ERD*, 6). What a wonderful sign, or sacrament as we explained earlier, Catholic pastoral care centers can be of the unfailing presence in the world of the sick of the Christ-Son who heals, of his God-Father who ongoingly creates, and of the Spirit of both who bears witness "that we are children of God, and if children then heirs, fellow heirs with Christ, provided we suffer with him in order that we may also be glorified with him" (Rom. 8:16–17). Paul pursues this thought, asking his Roman disciples, "Who shall separate us from the love of God? Shall tribulation, or distress, or persecution, or famine, or nakedness, or peril?" His answer is firm: "No, in all these things we are more than conquerors through him who loved us" (Rom. 8:35–37). So it is too with the sick who, nurtured by Catholic pastoral care, acknowledge the abiding presence of God within them even in their sickness and imminent death.

COLLABORATION TENSIONS

Revision in the 2018 *ERD* largely focuses on part 6, "Collaborative Arrangements with Other Health Care Organizations and Providers." Catholic health care institutions are entering into such collaborative arrangements with non-Catholic ones for three reasons: to ensure their survival in a very competitive health care market, to contribute more to the common health care good, and to extend their witness to Christ's healing ministry to an ever-larger population. A statement in the CDF's "Principles" is relevant here: "It is precisely the decisions of individuals that determine the identity and moral character of an institution."[16] In our day, the sexual abuse scandal in the Catholic Church and its cover-up by many bishops has led to a loss of trust in the authority not only of *individual* bishops who committed or covered up sexual abuse but also of the episcopal *office* itself and its ability to exercise credible authority on religious and moral matters. The revised *ERD* has made no effort to confront this situation.

Catholic health care institutions are necessarily entering into collaborative arrangements with non-Catholic hospitals to preserve Catholic ministry, influence, and witness. This collaboration inevitably raises a traditional Catholic moral question: Is it moral to cooperate with health care institutions that are performing medical procedures that the Catholic Church deems immoral—abortion, contraception, direct sterilization, physician-assisted suicide, for instance? It is significant that it is this question that so troubled the USCCB that it submitted a list of questions (*dubia*) to the CDF seeking guidance in general on collaborative relationships with non-Catholic health care institutions and in particular on collaboration in immoral procedures. We addressed the question, the CDF's response, and the USCCB's integration of its response in the revised *ERD* in chapter 6.

The response that guides collaborative relationships between Catholic and non-Catholic health care institutions focuses on bishops' ultimate authority to determine whether such relationships abide by natural law, Catholic moral teaching, and canon law; avoid scandal; and promote the Church's witness. The *ERD* focuses on absolute norms and the institution, patient, and health care professionals' obedience to these norms. As we argue, however, Church witness should focus not on absolute norms but on the foundational principle of Catholic health care, Jesus' healing ministry. The *ERD*'s emphasis on adherence to absolute norms as stated in its primary concern for collaborative relationships rather than Jesus' healing ministry as the foundation of all Catholic and non-Catholic health care highlights the tensions and shortcomings of the *ERD* anthropologically, methodologically, ecclesiologically, and pastorally. We conclude, then, with suggestions for future revisions of the *ERD* that include correctives to these tensions.

PROPOSALS TO ADDRESS TENSIONS IN THE *ERD*

Drawing extensively from Pope Francis and based on our proposed holistic anthropology, methodology, communion-synodal ecclesiology, emphasis on pastoral ministry and collaboration grounded in Christ's healing ministry, we propose the following for a revised *ERD*. First and foremost, the general introduction to the current *ERD* summarizes the essence of Catholic health care: "The mystery of Christ casts light on every facet of Catholic health care: to see Christian love as the animating principle of health care; to see healing and compassion as a continuation of Christ's mission; to see suffering as a participation in the redemptive power of Christ's passion, death, and resurrection; and to see death, transformed by the resurrection, as an opportunity for a final act of communion with Christ" (*ERD*, 6). The animating principle of Catholic health care should be guided by Jesus' healing ministry, the commandment to love God with one's whole mind, body, and soul, and to love one's neighbor as oneself, and to "go and do likewise" in imitation of Christ. This principle should animate and guide Catholic health care institutions, their health care professionals, staff, and administrators, and collaborative relationships.

Second, human dignity is foundational to Catholic health care. As we have demonstrated extensively, there is pluralism in Catholic definitions of human dignity and, based on those plural definitions, pluralism in the norms or directives that facilitate and do not frustrate realizing human dignity. The directives must account for this pluralism, especially in sexual health care issues, and reinstate the authority and inviolability of a well-informed conscience as the essential component of human dignity. No edition of the *ERD* has recognized the authority and inviolability of conscience emphasized at the Second Vatican Council in *Gaudium et Spes* and *Dignitatis Humanae* and re-emphasized in Pope Francis's anthropology. The *ERD* subordinates the authority and inviolability of patient conscience to the health care institution and, ultimately, to the authority of the bishop. This usurpation reflects an assault on human dignity and a violation of justice. Reinstating the authority of patient conscience introduces a fundamental requirement to shift the *ERD* from a focus on absolute norms and intrinsically evil acts to principled guidelines for forming consciences and allowing consciences, through the process of discernment, to make moral judgments regarding health care that are informed by Catholic teaching in dialogue with other sources of ethical knowledge. This process of discernment may lead to health care decisions that coincide with Catholic moral teaching, but it may also lead to decisions that disagree with those teachings. The animating principle of Catholic health care, Christ's healing ministry, is the supreme principle that should guide treatment of patients. Respecting decisions of conscience is part of that treatment.

Third, Pope Francis's emphasis on the virtues in *Amoris Laetitia* and the virtue of care in *Laudato Si'* should transition the *ERD* from a focus on specific directives and absolute norms to a focus on principles to guide patients as primary decision-makers and health care professionals as secondary decision-makers to responsible decisions of conscience given the particular historical, contextual, cultural, relational, and spiritual particularities of each individual. An example of such a principle to guide reproductive decisions is taken from the "Ethical Guidelines for Catholic Health Care Institutions": "Health care institutions are involved in aiding spouses to implement their procreative choices. In performing this service they should encourage responsible parenthood, which includes an openness to children, the appropriate limitation of conception when called for, and proper care of existing children."[17] The formulation of this guideline reflects the principle and virtue methodological approach of Pope Francis in comparison to the act-focus, absolute approach of the *ERD*. Pope Francis notes that natural methods of fertility regulation "are to be promoted" (*AL*, 222). Ultimately, the couple must decide how to realize responsible parenthood on the basis of an informed conscience, which is "the most secret core and sanctuary of a person" (*AL*, 222; *GS*, 16). Francis dedicates chapter 4 to a reflection on the virtue of love and its corresponding virtues. This is a crucial methodological shift at the heart of his new pastoral methods and can serve to shift the focus in the revised *ERD* from one on rules and laws to one on virtuous discernment and the prudential judgment of an informed conscience.

Fourth, there are several areas in the *ERD* that need to be revised, expanded on, or included in light of the anthropological, methodological, and ecclesiological critique of the *ERD* we have offered. We conclude with an overview of those areas.

Environment and Climate Change

Climate change is the greatest existential threat facing humanity and endangering its health. Pope Francis has warned what we all must surely know, that "time is running out!" The ecological crisis "threatens the very future of the human family" and "the climate crisis requires our decisive action here and now."[18] His encyclical on the ecological crisis, *Laudato Si'*, which documents the crisis with scientific evidence, details its devastating consequences for humanity, especially the poor, and calls for ecological conversion. This crisis has been largely ignored by the USCCB as a body and individual bishops in their dioceses. The World Health Organization recently issued a study that concludes, "No single country is adequately protecting children's health, their environment and their futures."[19] A comprehensive study of official columns written by every ordinary bishop in official publications from all 178 US Catholic dioceses revealed that between 2014 and 2019 less than 1 percent of 12,085 columns mention "climate change" or "global warming."[20] There is nothing in the revised *ERD* addressing the environmental crisis and its impact on health and health care. In its most recent meeting in November 2019, the USCCB repeated that abortion is the preeminent issue facing society and the issue that Catholics must prioritize. Cardinal Daniel DiNardo, its outgoing president, commented that climate change is an important but not urgent issue. Such episcopal response, or lack thereof, to climate change; its devastating impact on humanity, especially the poor and vulnerable; and its implications for Catholic health care, we believe, is unconscionable. Any revised version of the *ERD* must treat this threat to the health of humanity and propose concrete measures for Catholic health care to address health issues caused by climate change, address specific health care needs of the poor as a result of climate change, and mandate ways in which Catholic health care institutions can reduce their carbon footprint so as to reduce their contribution to the escalating crisis.[21] These, as much as abortion, we suggest, are genuinely pro-life issues.

Race

In the "Ethical Guidelines for Catholic Health Care Institutions," there is an explicit guideline focusing on race: "Minority races have suffered deeply at the hands of our society. The same is often true in Catholic health care institutions, both with regard to employees and patients. Catholic institutions should play a leading and aggressive role in redressing this imbalance, especially with regard to opportunities for advancement and respect for the dignity of persons."[22] A 2019 Centers for Disease Control and Prevention report released the results of a 2007–16 study on pregnancy-related mortality in the United States with disturbing conclusions. It concluded that the pregnancy-related mortality ratio (PRMR) for black and American Indian women older than thirty years of age was four to five times higher than for white women of a similar age. PRMR for black women with at least a college degree was 5.2 times higher than their white female counterparts. Even allowing for educational levels, this data highlights a crucial racial disparity in health care for pregnant women.[23]

The United States leads the developed world in PRMR.[24] In addition, life expectancy in the United States varies by race. In 2017 the average lifespan for Hispanics and Latinos was 81.8 years, for whites it was 78.6 years, and for Blacks it was 74.9 years.[25] There are other health disparities by race that indicate systemic racism in the United States and in the health care industry, and Catholic institutions not only are not immune from but may also contribute to this racism. Even though the USCCB has attempted to address the issue of racism through pastoral letters, those letters have been critiqued socially, culturally, theologically, and ethically.[26] There is a sense of institutional *scotosis* or moral blind spot with the USCCB when it comes to addressing race in pastorals specifically designed for that purpose. Although the *ERD* calls Catholic health care to advocate for and serve people who are socially marginalized and particularly vulnerable to discrimination, including "the poor; the uninsured and the underinsured; children and the unborn; single parents; the elderly; those with incurable diseases and chemical dependencies; racial minorities; immigrants and refugees," it lacks concrete proposals for doing so in light of the social scientific data that highlights the systemic discrimination and structural sin that perpetuates that discrimination. Especially during a period of heightened racial tensions in the United States, spawned in large part by the Trump administration and white nationalist movements, and the ongoing social, cultural, and political turmoil these tensions create and how they impact health outcomes for racial minorities, such an addition is crucial. The "Ethical Guideline" on race is perhaps more relevant today than it was in 1984. The *ERD* should be more deeply attentive to the signs of the times documented by the social sciences and more responsive to the needs of these populations. This is especially true in our day with increases in refugee and immigration populations and the phenomenon now being called the "browning of America."

Immigrants, Refugees, and Minorities

The US Census Bureau predicts that in 2044, the non-Hispanic white population will no longer make up a majority of the US population. The demographics are shifting, yet there is little acknowledgment of this shift in the *ERD* and no consideration of what it means for Catholic and non-Catholic health care delivery. In chapter 3 we noted the "white space" of American Catholic health care. It is past time to ask about the specific health care needs of immigrant, refugee, and minority populations and how Catholic health care can address these needs. Two examples illustrate the importance of this question. First, access to health care, especially in poor communities, is an essential component of Catholic social teaching. In our own city of Omaha, Nebraska, a Catholic hospital that served the largely low-income African American and Hispanic communities moved several miles west to merge with an existing Catholic hospital, and a substantially downsized Catholic clinic was constructed to replace it. Such a move risks reducing access to health care for poor and vulnerable communities and does nothing to promote a vision of solidarity with the poor that is at the heart of Catholic social teaching and that is stated specifically in the *ERD*. Financial expediency is often a prime reason dictating Catholic decisions about health care and, while we have no doubt that finances are important, so too are foundational Catholic social principles.

A second example is the reality of female genital mutilation or circumcision, especially among African Muslim populations. Many of these women have undergone circumcision in their home countries or have illegally been subjected to it in the United States. A question for Catholic health care institutions is whether, when pregnant women who have undergone this procedure give birth in Catholic health care facilities, these women should be reinfibulated after giving birth. Not to do so may jeopardize their social standing with their spouses, families, and communities; to do so may violate their physical, emotional, and mental health. The medical community has no decisive guidelines on what to do in this situation, even though it is increasing in frequency due to a growing refugee population in the United States. The *ERD* could function as a visionary leader to address these and other health care, social, and cultural ethical issues confronting an immigrant population. It could demonstrate a sensitivity to diversity and promote a balanced response that witnesses to diversity and seeks to extend Christ's healing ministry to immigrant populations.

Technological Developments and Their Implications for the *ERD*

The *ERD* tends to ignore current technological developments and the ethical challenges they pose for health care in general and Catholic health care in specific. It addresses technology in relation to reproduction, end-of-life issues, and collaborative relationships. There is a reference in the section on collaborative relationships to "medical technologies and expertise that greatly enhance the quality of care" (*ERD*, 23) that ensue in such collaborations, and there is a reaffirmation of Catholic norms prohibiting the use of technology in the case of reproductive technologies and permitting informed decision-making by a patient or designated surrogate in end-of-life issues, but there is no effort to come to ethical terms with newer and advanced technologies. CRISPR, for instance, the technology to edit genes and effect the phenotype and genotype of an individual that can be transmitted to future generations, cries out to be addressed in the *ERD*.[27] So too does rapidly advancing artificial intelligence (AI). Pope Francis highlights this need. AI, he notes, "touches the very threshold of the biological specificity and spiritual difference of the human being."

He warns that AI may be "socially dangerous," threatening the common good in general and health care in specific, casting "a dangerous spell" by moving toward a more "technologized" rather than a "technology humanized" anthropology.[28] As technology in health care rapidly develops, there is an urgent need to revise and update the *ERD* in light of these developments. Before the 2018 edition, the previous edition was published in 2009, and the only serious revisions in the 2018 edition address collaborative relationships between Catholic and non-Catholic health care institutions and focus on the bishop's authority to interpret and apply the *ERD*. Such limited revision, we suggest, is a dereliction of bishops' teaching duty.

Sex and Gender

As we become more culturally and ethically sensitive to the fundamental equality of women and men, the Church needs to be more explicit in its prophetic witness that recognizes this equality and its ethical implications for Catholic health care. This impacts several dimensions of Catholic institutions. First, there must be an emphasis on just and equal pay for men and women in the health care profession. The sociological data in 2019 indicate that women, on average, are paid $0.79 for each dollar men are paid.[29] Catholic health care institutions are not immune to this disparity. Catholic social justice teaching requires that some mention be made in the *ERD* of just wages and the possibility of unions to ensure just wages. This would be helpful in promoting a Christian witness for gender justice. Second, as transgender people feel increasingly able to live openly in our society, the *ERD* needs to engage health care issues specific to their reality anthropologically and ethically. Anthropologically, it needs to embrace "Male and Female He Created Them" and its invitation to dialogue about sex *and* gender and not conflate the two in ethical responses to transgender people and their requests for transitioning therapies. As we argued throughout this book, the *ERD* too often reflects a reductionist biological ontology and anthropology rather than a holistic and personalist anthropology. This anthropological shift will require thoughtful theological and ethical dialogue on sex and gender, their interrelationship and not conflation, and how to care for and treat gender dysphoria in Catholic institutions and the non-Catholic institutions that collaborate with them.

Poverty

Pope Francis has emphasized climate change and poverty as the most pressing issues facing humanity. When asked if the Church should consider a change in its absolute prohibition of the use of condoms to prevent the spread of HIV/ AIDS, the pope responded that the question seemed too small: "I think the morality of the Church on this point finds itself in a dilemma: is it the fifth or the sixth commandment? To defend life, or is the sexual relation open to life? But this is not the problem." The first problem in Africa, and indeed worldwide, he said, is much bigger and more complex than the use of condoms. The first problem is the reality of "denutrition, the exploitation of people, slave labor, lack of drinking water."[30] Condom use may or may not address a part of the human problem, but the greater problem is systemic social injustice and violations of human dignity throughout the world. Catholic social teaching is the Catholic Church's best keep secret, but thanks to Pope Francis it is now getting more exposure and emphasis.

In his writings, Francis emphasizes "the growing gap in healthcare possibilities" due to economic inequities. "Access to healthcare risks being more dependent on individuals' economic resources than on their actual need for treatment." With regard to health care and end-of-life issues, he notes, "Increasingly sophisticated and costly treatments are available to ever more limited and privileged segments of the population, and this raises questions about the sustainability of healthcare delivery and about what might be called a systemic tendency toward growing inequality in health care."[31] We encourage the USCCB in its next revision of the *ERD* to be more emphatic about poverty and its impact on the lives, health, and human dignity of all people. It should take a more holistic approach to how poverty and economics affect ethical decisions, especially the reproductive decisions of poor women of color. Not to engage the impact of poverty on health care and the relationship between gender and poverty risks reducing Catholic social teaching and its emphasis on poverty to a peripheral issue that does not adequately consider the concerns of poor people.

The question of poverty and access to health care could be expanded to consider issues of the growing disparity between rich and poor and the ever-growing cost of health care and health insurance. Highlighting the exorbitant cost of prescription drugs and the tragic choices many people have to make between purchasing and taking their full medical prescriptions or paying for food and housing is a foundational and common social justice issue in the United States. These concerns surrounding poverty, social justice, and the cost of health care should be preeminent concerns among bishops and should be addressed in the *ERD*.

Law, Policy, and Religious Freedom

One final issue, which is not addressed in the *ERD* but has occupied a great deal of the USCCB's time, energy, and financial resources, is the issue of religious liberty in relation to law, public policy, and health care. The USCCB has made religious liberty a preeminent issue for the Catholic Church in the twenty-first-century United States. It has spent innumerable resources fighting the contraceptive mandate of the Affordable Care Act, writing amicus curiae briefs on issues surrounding homosexuality and gender identity to fight nondiscrimination legislation and to protect the consciences and decisions of for-profit private corporations like Hobby Lobby not to provide contraceptives in their insurance plans. The USCCB has gradually expanded its advocacy for religious freedom, from exemption from what it perceives to be unjust laws to the repeal of just laws.

The USCCB opposes legislation and public policy that violate Catholic teachings, largely related to sexual ethical issues such as the ACA's contraceptive mandate and non-discrimination legislation related to homosexual orientation or gender identity. Such opposition cites religious liberty and freedom of conscience to argue for exemption from or the repeal of laws already enacted and the rejection of laws under legislative consideration. Douglas Laycock notes that "reliance on a distinction between just laws that violate the tenets of a particular faith, for which the solution is an exemption, and unjust laws for which the only solution is repeal" is the most problematic aspect of the USCCB's "Statement on Religious Liberty."[32] Seeking an exemption, prevention, or repeal under the auspices of religious liberty is to confuse the argument about moral issues and the argument about religious liberty.[33]

The USCCB cites Pope Benedict in defense of religious liberty in its "Statement." "Many of you," Benedict stated, "have pointed out that concerted efforts have been made to deny the right of conscientious objection on the part of Catholic individuals and institutions with regard to *cooperation in intrinsically evil practices.*"[34] Among those intrinsically evil practices in the judgment of the Church and named in the *ERD* are contraception, abortion, euthanasia, direct sterilization, and physician-assisted suicide. David Hollenbach and Thomas Shannon note, however, that the "Catholic moral tradition has long stressed that civil law should be founded on moral values but need not seek to abolish all immoral activities in society."[35] The bishops are free to assert in a moral argument seeking to regulate life in the public domain that Catholic and non-Catholic health care institutions should not perform acts they consider to be intrinsically evil.[36] Should such a moral argument, however, be codified in legislation? It is one thing to claim an exemption for a religious institution from a just law on the basis of conscientious objection to the moral contents of the law, it is quite another to seek repeal or prevention of a law based on that objection. The bishops have not made this distinction in their resistance to the contraceptive mandate and seek to make Catholic moral imperatives on sexuality legal national imperatives. They claim that the ACA contraceptive mandate is an "unjust law" because it promotes immoral sexual conduct and immoral regulation of fertility. They note that it is essential to understand the distinction between conscientious objection and an unjust law. Conscientious objection applies to a just law and seeks a religious exemption from it, but "an unjust law is 'no law at all;' it cannot be obeyed, and therefore one does not seek relief from it, but rather its repeal."[37] Laycock notes correctly that "the difference between exemption and repeal is the difference between seeking religious liberty for Catholic institutions and seeking to impose Catholic moral teaching on the nation" and, we add, non-Catholic health care institutions.[38]

Although recent editions of the *ERD* have been consistent in their teachings on intrinsically evil acts that should be prohibited in Catholic and non-Catholic institutions and should not be legalized, such as abortion, euthanasia, and physician-assisted suicide, the majority of lay Catholics do not accept those teachings. The fact that the majority of Catholic faithful do not accept Catholic teaching on the immorality of these acts is not a moral argument, for morality is not determined by majority consensus. The burden of proof, however, is on the Church to make a compelling argument to convince Catholics that its teachings are true. Hollenbach and Shannon suggest that "the church should not ask the state [or non-Catholic health care institutions] to do what it has not been able to convince its own members to do."[39] The Church should not ask the state or a health care institution to enforce a law, policy, or teaching that it cannot convince the majority of its own members to accept. The burden of proof is on the Church to demonstrate that such acts are in fact, as it claims, destructive of human dignity and cannot serve "the good of the person or society." So far it has not offered a compelling argument for many of those assertions. An unproven assertion should not be advanced or allowed as the basis for an abuse of religious freedom aimed at preventing or repealing law, policy, or practice and imposing the Church's morally questionable doctrine on the broader society.

In the USCCB's "Statement," borrowing Martin Luther King's phrase, the bishops write that they want to be the "conscience of the state." They seek to extend Catholic moral teaching beyond a religious exemption from a just law to the prevention or repeal of a law they deem unjust. While the Catholic Church teaches that euthanasia, abortion, and contraception are morally wrong, the majority of Americans consider them morally acceptable. Some even consider them to be a human right. As William Galston correctly notes, "The Bishops make no effort to understand why their antagonists think that justice requires what the Catholic hierarchy thinks it forbids."[40] To claim a religious exemption from a just law is one thing; to claim repeal or prevention of an unjust law is quite another and raises both the legal and the ethical bars high. The bishops have every right to teach a moral position and to seek to protect religious institutions from participation in what they perceive as immoral activity, but they do not have a right to seek to impose their moral teachings legislatively or in terms of institutional policy on a pluralistic society. That would be akin to proselytizing and a violation of many well-informed consciences.

CONCLUSION

We conclude our critical analysis of the *ERD* in particular and Catholic health care teaching in general with a statement from Pope Francis that summarizes well what we have proffered in this commentary as a corrective for the *ERD*.

> We cannot insist only on issues related to abortion, gay marriage and the use of contraceptive methods. . . . The church's pastoral ministry cannot be obsessed with the transmission of a disjointed multitude of doctrines to be imposed insistently. We have to find a new balance; otherwise even the moral edifice of the Church [and Catholic health care] is likely to fall like a house of cards, losing the freshness and fragrance of the Gospel.[41]

We have taken Pope Francis's warning seriously and, drawing largely on his papal writings, have proposed a new balance. This new balance is a revised anthropology, methodology, and ecclesiology that reflects Francis's concern for pastoral ministry and that seeks to revise the *ERD* into a more comprehensive, compassionate, ethical, and legal document that extends Christ's healing ministry to all, especially to the poor and vulnerable.

SUGGESTED READING

Keenan, James F. "What Is Pope Francis's Effect on Health Care?" *America*, May 18, 2018. https://www.americamagazine.org/politics-society/2018/05/18/what-pope-francis-effect-health-care.

Lysaught, M. Therese, and Michael McCarthy, eds. *Catholic Bioethics and Social Justice: The Praxis of US Health Care in a Globalized World*. Collegeville, MN: Liturgical Press, 2018.

Salzman, Todd A., and Michael G. Lawler. *The Sexual Person: Toward a Renewed Catholic Anthropology*. Washington, DC: Georgetown University Press, 2008.

NOTES

1. McCormick, *Health and Medicine*, 160.

2. Pew Research Center, "In U.S., Decline of Christianity Continues at Rapid Pace," October 17, 2019, available at https://www.pewforum.org/2019/10/17/in-u-s

-decline-of-christianity-continues-at-rapid-pace/. See Ken Briggs, "The Laity Hold the Key to Reforming the Church," *National Catholic Reporter*, December 3, 2018, available at https://www.ncronline.org/news/opinion/ncr-today/laity-hold-key-reforming -church; PRRI, "National Catholic Reporter Highlights PRRI Data in Exploration of American Catholics," December 13, 2013, available at https://www.prri.org/spot light/national-catholic-reporter-highlights-prri-data-in-exploration-of-american-cath olics/; Pew Research Center, "Americans See Catholic Clergy Sex Abuse as an Ongo-ing Problem," June 11, 2019, available at https://www.pewforum.org/2019/06/11/ameri cans-see-catholic-clergy-sex-abuse-as-an-ongoing-problem/.

3. Document available at http://www.vatican.va/content/francesco/en/apost_exhor tations/documents/papa-francesco_esortazione-ap_20200202_querida-amazonia.html.

4. See Cahill, "Catholic Sexual Ethics," 145–46; Johnson, "Disembodied 'Theology of the Body,'" 11–17; Margaret Farley, *Just Love: A Framework for Christian Sexual Ethics* (New York: Continuum, 2006).

5. Karol Wojtyla, *Love and Responsibility* (Boston: Pauline Books and Media, 2013), 229–30, 53.

6. See also The Pontifical Council for the Family, "Family, Marriage and 'De Facto' Unions," January 11, 2001, 8, available at http://www.vatican.va/roman_curia/pontifical _councils/family/documents/rc_pc_family_doc_20001109_de-facto-unions_en.html: "According to this ideology [of gender], being a man or a woman is not determined fun-damentally by sex but by culture. Therefore, the very bases of the family and interpersonal relationships are attacked." According to this statement, biological sex and not cultural gender is the foundation for interpersonal relationships.

7. See Salzman and Lawler, *Sexual Person*, ch. 2.

8. Pentin, "Cardinal Parolin," *National Catholic Register*.

9. McCormick, *Health and Medicine in the Catholic Tradition*, 11.

10. Catholic Health Association, "Report on a Theological Dialogue on the Principle of Cooperation," *Health Progress* (November–December 2007): 68–69, available at https:// www.chausa.org/docs/default-source/health-progress/report-on-a-theological-dia logue-on-the-principle-of-cooperation-pdf.pdf?sfvrsn=2.

11. Schneiders, "Religion and Spirituality," 4–5.

12. "Primary Health Care Now More than Ever," World Health Organization, 2008, 43, available at http://www.who.int/whr/2008/en/.

13. Dietrich Von Hildebrand, *Marriage* (London: Longmans, 1939), v.

14. Pontifical Council for Pastoral Assistance to Health Care Workers, *Charter for Health Care*, 145, cited in David Albert Jones, "Gender Reassignment Surgery: A Catholic Bioeth-ical Analysis," *Theological Studies* 79, no. 2 (2018): 314–38, at 317n10. Jones notes that the new edition of the charter removed any reference to transsexual medicine or surgery.

15. See Jones, "Gender Reassignment Surgery," 320–21; and Susannah Cornwall, "'State of Mind' versus 'Concrete Set of Facts': The Contrasting of Transgender and Intersex in Church Documents on Sexuality," *Theology & Sexuality* 15, no. 1 (2009): 7–28.

16. Congregation for the Doctrine of the Faith, "Some Principles," 338.

17. McCormick, *Health and Medicine in the Catholic Tradition*, 12.

18. "Address of His Holiness Pope Francis to Participants at the Meeting Promoted by the Dicastery for Promoting Integral Human Development on the Theme: The Energy Transition & Care of Our Common Home," June 14, 2019, available at http://www.vatican.va/content/francesco/en/speeches/2019/june/documents/papa-francesco_20190614_compagnie-petrolifere.html.

19. "World Failing to Provide Children with a Healthy Life and a Climate Fit for Their Future: WHO-UNICEF-Lancet," World Health Organization, February 19, 2020, available at https://www.who.int/news-room/detail/19-02–2020-world-failing-to-provide-children-with-a-healthy-life-and-a-climate-fit-for-their-future-who-unicef-lancet.

20. Sabrina Danielsen, Daniel R. DiLeo, and Emily Burke, "The Duty to Teach: U.S. Bishops, Climate Change, and Catholic Social Teaching," paper presented at the Society for the Scientific Study of Religion 2019 Annual Meeting, Saint Louis, October 26, 2019.

21. For extensive resources on climate change and Catholic health care, see "Climate Change and Catholic Health Care: A Matter of Faith, Hope and Charity," Catholic Health Association of the United States, available at https://www.chausa.org/environment/climate-change.

22. McCormick, *Health and Medicine*, 10–11.

23. "Racial and Ethnic Disparities Continue in Pregnancy-Related Deaths," CDC, September 5, 2019, available at https://www.cdc.gov/media/releases/2019/p0905-racial-ethnic-disparities-pregnancy-deaths.html.

24. Nina Martin and Renee Montagne, "U.S. Has the Worst Rate of Maternal Deaths in the Developed World," National Public Radio, May 12, 2017, https://www.npr.org/2017/05/12/528098789/u-s-has-the-worst-rate-of-maternal-deaths-in-the-developed-world.

25. "Life Expectancy at Birth, by Sex and Race and Hispanic Origin: United States, 2007–2017," CDC, https://www.cdc.gov/nchs/data/hus/2018/fig01.pdf.

26. USCCB, "Open Wide Our Hearts"; USCCB, "Brothers and Sisters to Us" (Washington, DC: US Catholic Bishops, 1979), available at http://www.usccb.org/issues-and-action/cultural-diversity/african-american/brothers-and-sisters-to-us.cfm; and USCCB, "Discrimination and Christian Conscience: A Statement by the Catholic Bishops of the United States," November 14, 1958, available at http://www.usccb.org/issues-and-action/cultural-diversity/african-american/resources/upload/Discrimination-Christian-Conscience-Nov-14-1958.pdf. See Bryan N. Massingale, *Racial Justice and the Catholic Church* (Maryknoll, NY: Orbis, 2010).

27. See Charles C. Camosy, "CRISPR Gene Technology Poses New Moral Questions," *Crux*, November 5, 2019, available at https://cruxnow.com/interviews/2019/11/crispr-gene-technology-poses-new-moral-questions/.

28. "Address of His Holiness Pope Francis to Participants in the Plenary Assembly of the Pontifical Academy of Life," February 25, 2019, available at http://www.vatican.va/content/francesco/en/speeches/2019/february/documents/papa-francesco_20190225_plenaria-accademia-vita.html.

29. Shahar Ziv, "3 Ways the Gender Pay Gap Is Even Bigger than You Think," *Forbes*,

July 11, 2019, available at https://www.forbes.com/sites/shaharziv/2019/07/11/gender-pay-gap-bigger-than-you-thnk/#28361b7c7d8a.

30. Gerard O'Connell, "Pope Francis on Paris Climate Change Summit: 'It's Either Now or Never,'" *America*, November 30, 2015, available at https://www.americamagazine.org/content/dispatches/popes-press-conference-flight-bangui-rome.

31. "Message of His Holiness Pope Francis to the Participants in the European Regional Meeting of the World Medical Association," November 7, 2017, available at http://w2.vatican.va/content/francesco/en/messages/pont-messages/2017/documents/papa-francesco_20171107_messaggio-monspaglia.html.

32. USCCB, "Our First, Most Cherished Liberty: Statement on Religious Liberty," 2012, available at http://www.usccb.org/issues-and-action/religious-liberty/our-first-most-cherished-liberty.cfm.

33. Douglas Laycock, "The Bishops & Religious Liberty," *Commonweal*, May 30, 2012, available at https://www.commonwealmagazine.org/bishops-religious-liberty.

34. USCCB, "Our First, Most Cherished Liberty."

35. David Hollenbach and Thomas Shannon, "A Balancing Act: Catholic Teaching on the Church's Rights—and the Rights of All," *America*, March 5, 2012, available at http://americamagazine.org/issue/5131/article/balancing-act.

36. Laycock, "Bishops & Religious Liberty."

37. USCCB, "Our First, Most Cherished Liberty."

38. Laycock, "Bishops & Religious Liberty."

39. Hollenbach and Shannon, "Balancing Act."

40. Laycock, "Bishops & Religious Liberty."

41. Pope Francis, "Message of His Holiness Pope Francis." See also James F. Keenan, "What Is Pope Francis's Effect on Health Care?" *America*, May 18, 2018, available at https://www.americamagazine.org/politics-society/2018/05/18/what-pope-francis-effect-health-care.

Index

About the Authors

Todd A. Salzman is the Amelia and Emil Graff Professor of Catholic Theology at Creighton University. He is married to Katy C. Salzman, and they have three children, Ian, Aaron, and Emily. He enjoys spending time with family and friends, traveling, hunting, and fishing.

Michael G. Lawler is a dean emeritus of Creighton University's Graduate School of Arts and Sciences and an emeritus Amelia and Emil Graff Professor of Catholic Theology at Creighton. He has held faculty appointments at St. Joseph College, Nairobi, Kenya, and Holy Ghost College, Dublin. He is married to Susan R. Hoffman, and they have three children, Michael, Anya, and David.

Together, they have published *The Sexual Person: Toward a Renewed Catholic Anthropology* (Georgetown, 2008); *Sexual Ethics: A Theological Introduction* (Georgetown, 2012); *The Church in the Modern World: Gaudium et Spes Then and Now* (Liturgical Press, 2014); *Virtue and Theological Ethics: Toward a Renewed Ethical Method* (Orbis, 2018); and *Introduction to Theological Ethics: Foundations and Applications* (Orbis, 2019). They have also published a number of scholarly articles in *Theological Studies, Heythrop Journal, Louvain Studies, Horizons, Irish Theological Quarterly,* and *America.*